Welcome to the premier edition of

Calix

International Journal of Flower Essence Therapy

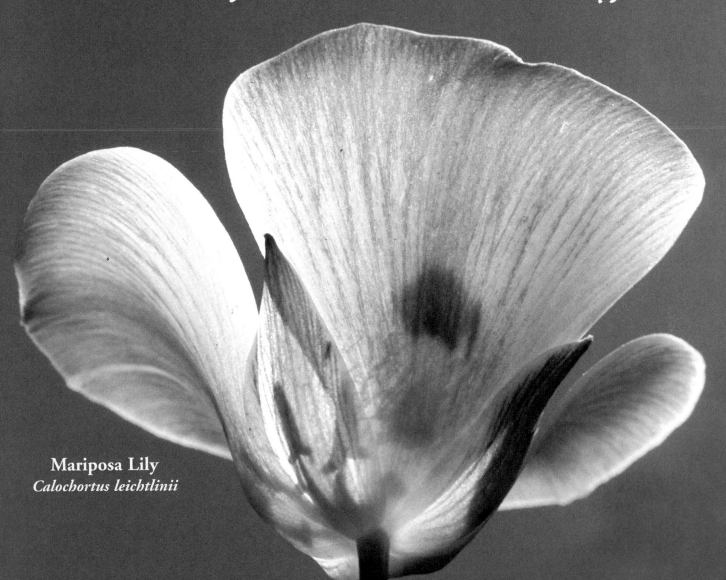

Mariposa Lily
Calochortus leichtlinii

Calix (ka'liks), *n*. A cup or chalice. See Calyx.

Calyx (ka'liks), *n*. (botany) the cup of a flower, a whorl of sepals collectively forming the outer floral envelope; enclosing and supporting the developing bud; usually green

In the quiet blossom's star
Flexed muscle of infinite receptivity
Often so overwhelmed with fullness
That the sunset's call to rest
Can hardly return to
Your wide-relaxed petals.

You, the firmness and fortitude
Of many worlds.
We are violent
And stay around longer.
But when, in which of our lives,
Will we finally open up and become receptive?

Rainer Maria Rilke, Sonnets to Orpheus

Star Tulip
Calochortus tolmiei

The name we have chosen for our new journal is rich with meaning. What is the essential nature of a cup? It is a form which can receive and enclose what is poured into it. Because of its receptive nature, it can also give of its contents; be poured out as nourishment. Certainly a cup is an ordinary and practical object, one we use in quite a utilitarian manner to satisfy our thirst. But when we think of it as a chalice, we consider that a cup can also be quite sacred, it can hold sacramental substance that nourishes both body and soul.

Similarly, the botanical description of a calyx can seem quite mundane; it is a technical term to describe the physical anatomy of a flower. But when we behold a plant as it metamorphoses through its stages of growth, we realize that the moment of becoming a calyx is quite extraordinary. This exquisite green structure of the plant is truly a sacred chalice; it is a container that holds the forces of the cosmos, so that the plant might become receptive to something higher. What we encounter in the plant at its moment of becoming a flower touches our soul with wondrous color, form, and fragrance; we sense that a gift from other worlds has appeared on earth. The poet, Rilke, expressed this truth in his *Sonnets to Orpheus*. (See poem on the facing page.)

From the perspective of our narrow ego, we humans may consider that we are "higher" than a flower. As Rilke suggests, certainly we wield more physical prowess and live a longer life. Yet, if we consider the flower with utter humility we might realize that the very purity and receptivity of the flower gives it a position of great strength in the spiritual world. Like Parsifal, who was changed when he beheld a field of flowers on Good Friday, medieval seekers of the Holy Grail sensed that the flower was teaching us something about the chalice possibilities of our own souls. Each flower reaches fulfillment with a kind of desire or "soul blood," that is absolutely pure and grace-filled.

Surely it was this same quest which impelled Dr. Edward Bach when he abandoned his prestigious position on Harley Street in London to return to the open fields of his Celtic ancestry, where his feet could "walk England's green and pleasant land."* There, an inspiration filled him — an exceptional understanding of healing that could not be attributed to his strict medical training. Dr. Bach realized that medicines could be made from flowers in "Nature's laboratory," by being present to the holy moment of each blossom in communion with the weaving elements and the cosmos. These unique preparations would have a profound ability to speak to the human soul; cleansing it of fear, greed, bitterness, separation—the myriad ways in which human desire falls short of what the flower gives in such a pure manner.

The **Flower Essence Society** now celebrates more than a quarter-century of service to the worldwide development of flower essence therapy. The purpose for launching this new journal is evocative of a **Calyx** – "an outer floral envelope that supports a developing bud." We intend that our publication be a container for supporting the pioneering efforts of this new healing modality by profiling many practitioners from around the world, including theoretical and professional research about plant science and flower essence therapy.

And we hope too, that this journal is a **Calix**. May it be received like a sacred chalice that pours its sustenance into the soul of each reader, giving new inspiration, insight and nourishment about flower essence therapy.

Patricia Kaminski, Editor

* the image of walking England's green and pleasant land can be found in William Blake's poem, "The New Jerusalem."

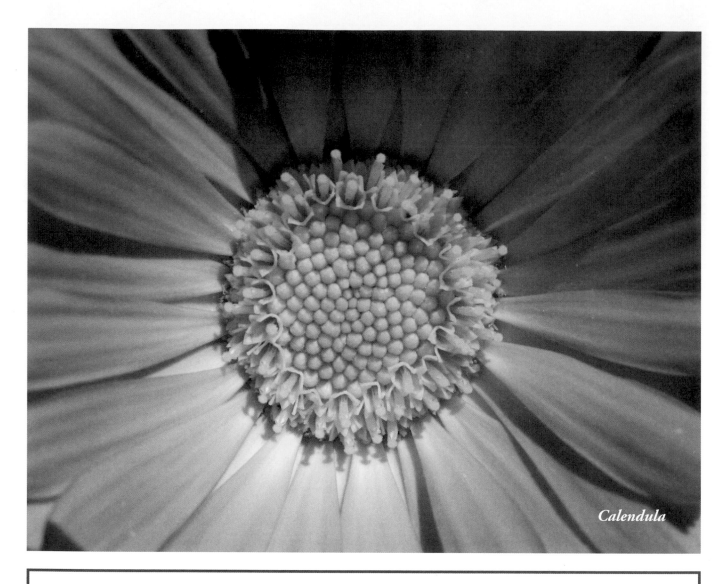

Calendula

Calix: International Journal of Flower Essence Therapy, Vol. 1

Published by the Flower Essence Society
a division of the non-profit educational and research organization, Earth-Spirit, Inc.

Executive Editor: Patricia Kaminski
Editorial Staff: Richard Katz, Jann Garitty, Patrick Warner, Alison Anderson, Sylvia Jordan
Graphic Design: Richard Katz, Jann Garitty   **Calix logo:** LeeAnn Brook
Flower and nature photography: Richard Katz, Julian Barnard, Getty Images

The poem "Entrance" on page 32, Copyright 2001 by Dana Giona
Reprinted from *Interrogations at Noon,* with the permission of Graywolf Press, Saint Paul, MN.

Flower Essence Society, PO Box 459, Nevada City, CA 95959 USA
www.flowersociety.org   800-736-9222   530-265-9163   fax: 530-265-0584

 Printed on recycled paper.
Cover is Primavera gloss, 80% recycled, 40% post-consumer, processed chlorine-free (New Leaf Paper Co.)

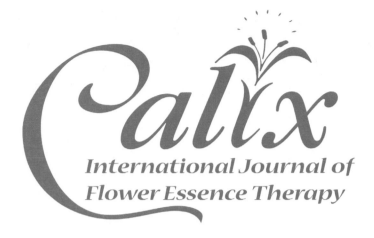

Calix
International Journal of Flower Essence Therapy

Table of Contents, Volume 1

Extending the Legacy of Dr. Edward Bach:

Flower Essence Therapy in the Twenty-First Century

by Patricia Kaminski

*The Daisy — or "day's eye" —
evokes a picture of the sun itself,
with its awake "eye" of light.*

A Debt of Gratitude to Dr. Bach

Contemporary practitioners of flower essence therapy owe a debt of gratitude to Dr. Edward Bach for his courage and genius as a healer. He stood virtually alone as a pioneer, teaching that feelings and thoughts within the human soul are intimately related to the overall condition of health. Dr. Bach understood that flowering plants have soul qualities that can be translated into extraordinary medicines, through a precise and reverent method of elemental preparation.

Do we honor Dr. Bach, as some of his successors contend, by letting his research stand as it existed in 1936, when he died? Each practitioner should feel free to answer this question according to personal choices and affinities. However, there is no definitive statement from Dr. Bach that he regarded his work as "complete" before his untimely death at age 50. It is true that he may have declared that he was "finished" with a phase of his investigations, but in reading Dr. Bach's biography we can see there were many such phases. The entire gesture of Dr. Bach's brief life was never static, but always open to new discoveries, and even a radical re-shaping of previously held views.

Dr. Bach's earliest inclination was to become a minister.[1] He chose a medical career, but only after working for a period of time in his father's brass foundry. He began as a surgeon (Casualty Medical Officer) in 1914, but then became much more interested in immunology, changing his specialty to become Assistant Bacteriologist at the London University School of Medicine. At the University Hospital, Dr. Bach developed his famous intestinal vaccines. Despite the success of these vaccines, he resigned from his position in 1918 and switched to a career in homeopathy at London Homeopathic Hospital. His oral vaccines were then developed as homeopathic nosodes and Dr. Bach became well-recognized in his profession. Yet by 1922, he resigned his post at the London Homeopathic Hospital to develop a private practice and to continue to investigate new ways of re-formulating his vaccines.

Then, in 1929, Dr. Bach abandoned all other methods of treatment in favor of three new herbal remedies he had developed. In 1930, he closed his lucrative Harley Street practice, distributed nearly all his possessions, and severed all of his ties in London to relocate in the Welsh countryside. There, he changed his three herbal remedies, re-formulating them as "flower remedies," and also added nine more essences to his repertoire.

Disease is in essence the result of conflict between Soul and Mind, and will never be eradicated except by spiritual and mental effort... No effort which is directed to the body alone can do more than superficially repair damage, and in this there is no cure, since the cause is still operative and may at any moment again demonstrate its presence in another form.

Dr. Edward Bach

In 1933, Dr. Bach published his research as the *Twelve Healers,* discarding various experimental remedies such as Pennywort (*Cotyledon umbilicus*),[2] Field Sow Thistle *(Sonchus arvensis)*[3] and Cypress *(Cupressus).*[4] Later that year, this same book was re-written to become *The Twelve Healers and the Four Helpers.* Next, in 1934, a second edition was published called *The Twelve Healers and the Seven Helpers.*

Then in 1935, only one year before his death, Dr. Bach doubled the size of his repertory, adding nineteen more flower essences. He gave the title *Twelve Healers and Other Remedies* to his third edition in 1936, just before he died on November 27, 1936. [5]

There is no question that we see a strong signature of continual investigation and openness to new approaches and reformulations, throughout Dr. Bach's entire life. Certainly, there is every reason to surmise that, had Dr. Bach's life continued beyond fifty short years, his work would have also grown and developed, including the addition of more remedies to his collection. Dr. Bach would no doubt have also continued to explore the philosophy and practice of soul healing as a foundation for flower essence therapy, beyond his early lectures and introductory essays.

Even if Dr. Bach had not chosen to develop his work further, we must recognize that collective wisdom in human culture has always evolved beyond the initial discoveries of any founder or pioneer. Indeed, Dr. Bach characterized his own work as a further step beyond that of his teacher, **Samuel Hahnemann.**[6] Perhaps the more important question is not *whether* new remedies and healing concepts can be developed, but *how* and *why.* What are the compelling moral reasons for doing so? Surely economic gain, fame, psychic glamour, or passing cultural fads cannot be genuine motives.

In this way, Dr. Bach is our teacher. His deep love for humanity and his tireless search to improve his methods of healing, even if that meant breaking the bounds of convention, are truly inspirational. Dr. Bach was a man of compassion and sensitivity who embraced the healing questions of his time. He began his career in charge of war beds for England's injured troops. There, he saw the agony, not only of the body, but also of the soul, in a world catastrophe of unspeakable cruelty, shattering the naïve optimism of the nineteenth century. The Great Depression, along with the rise of Nazism and Fascism in the 30s, brought widespread hopelessness and anxiety to all of humanity.

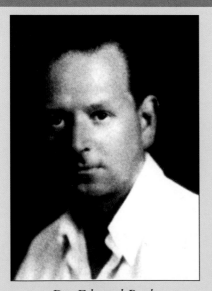

Dr. Edward Bach

Suffering is a corrective to point out a lesson which by other means we have failed to grasp, and never can it be eradicated until that lesson is learnt.

Dr. Edward Bach

It was during this time of deepest anguish — truly a soul "depression" within the whole of world culture — that Dr. Bach's 38 remedies were developed. Is it any wonder that the majority of them deal with despondency, loneliness, despair, mental torture, emotional constriction and fear?

All of these soul conditions continue to confront world culture, and Dr. Bach's flower remedies are as relevant today, as they were seven decades ago. However, the late twentieth century and early twenty-first century have brought new soul conditions and new challenges to our awareness. Examples include: the changing identity of masculine and feminine, spiritual emergence and heightened psychic sensitivity, a deeper recognition of the human shadow and how it must be healed, the role of creativity and individuality in soul development, the necessity of finding right livelihood and soul destiny in professional work, and the need for the human soul to establish a conscious relationship to Nature at a time when encroaching technology and urbanization threaten to annihilate such an awareness.

Building on Dr. Bach's Foundation

Dr. Bach laid a vital foundation for the new healing modality of flower essence therapy, yet the edifice could not be completed in those seven short years of work from 1929 to 1936. The need to build a more complete structure for flower essence therapy inspired Richard Katz to begin his research in 1977-78, joined by his wife and professional colleague, Patricia Kaminski in 1980. Through affiliation with numerous practitioners around the world, the work of the *Flower Essence Society* now spans a quarter-century of research. This research effort is not intended as a replacement, but rather an extension of the pioneering work of Dr. Bach, in three important areas:

1) The **development of a healing paradigm** for flower essence therapy through worldwide case research with practitioners. The goal is to develop a professional therapy that incorporates emerging knowledge from modern depth psychology, holistic health, and many paths of soul-spiritual wisdom.
2) **Advancement of a living science of Nature** with the objective of establishing a spiritual-scientific understanding for how qualities of plants translate into the healing properties of flower essences.
3) **Investigation and clinical documentation of new flower essences** to meet soul conditions that reflect the unique healing issues challenging modern humanity.

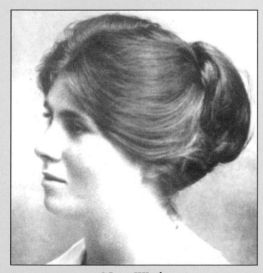

Nora Weeks

There were two great interests in his [Dr. Bach's] life — overwhelming compassion for all who suffered, whether human being, bird or beast, and love for Nature, for her trees and plants. These two combined to lead him to the knowledge of the healing that he sought.

Nora Weeks, companion of Dr. Bach and Director of the Bach Centre until her death in 1978

A Soul-Based Paradigm for Flower Essence Therapy

In the cultural context of the early 1930s, there was little support or understanding of Dr. Bach's ground-breaking therapeutic approach. Psychotherapy had only recently been introduced and was not yet widely practiced. Contemporary medical research largely discounted the role of psychosomatic factors in physical disease. It was only in 1936, the year of Dr. Bach's death, that **Hans Selye** (1907-1982) published his first findings on stress as a factor in disease.[7] Furthermore, the understanding of the human soul as a distinct entity separate from both body and spirit — though intimately related to both — was not yet fully articulated. The word "soul" was mostly regarded as an obscure theological concept, and esoteric teachings for soul development were closely guarded by small, secretive groups, like the Masonic Lodge, of which Dr. Bach himself was a member.

Richard Katz and Patricia Kaminski realized that in the decades since Dr. Bach died, cultural advances have provided an entirely new context for flower essence therapy. For example, the development of humanistic and transpersonal psychology, based on the hierarchy of needs of **Abraham Maslow**[8] (1908–1970), emphasizes self-actualization as a higher goal of human potential than behavioral adjustment to cultural norms or expectations. The Swiss psychiatrist **Carl Jung**[9] (1875–1961) described and documented the immense territory of the soul. He established that the "shadow" and other unconscious aspects of the human identity should not be repressed or simply regarded as "negative," but rather they should be redeemed, transformed and integrated into the whole of the Self.

Jung's pioneering research especially complements Dr. Bach's. Just as we can find key archetypal qualities in flowers, Jung showed that those archetypes also exist independently in the human soul, presenting rich possibilities for alchemical transformation. Building on the archetypal vision of Dr. Jung, the Italian psychiatrist **Roberto Assagioli**[10] (1888–1974) founded a school of psychotherapy called **Psychosynthesis**, in which he posited a core spiritual self as the guiding principle for the various sub-personalities, or archetypal qualities within one's being. **Viktor E. Frankl**[11] (1905-1997) validated his own theories about the soul's health through several years of incarceration in Nazi prison camps. His **Logotherapy** champi-

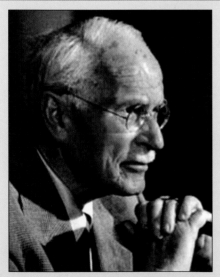

Dr. Carl Gustav Jung

As a plant produces its flower, so the psyche creates its symbols.

No archetype can be reduced to a simple formula. ... It is a vessel which can never empty and never fill. ... It persists through the ages and requires interpreting ever anew.

Dr. Carl Gustav Jung

ons the essential freedom of the soul to find spiritual meaning in life despite all external circumstances — teaching that each human being has not only a right, but a responsibility, to realize potential and find purpose in life.

In addition to these four early luminaries, there are many other contributors to modern psychotherapy, whose casework and theoretical models continue to verify the enormous arena of the human soul and its impact on both body and spirit. It is beyond the scope of this particular essay to cover all of these noteworthy contributions in detail. What is important for the purposes of this article, is to recognize the remarkable progress of psychotherapeutic healing and philosophy since Dr. Bach's life. The quest to understand the role of the human soul in healing is one that is intimately related to Dr. Bach's early vision, and yet has also evolved significantly since that time.

Beginning in the late 1970s, the *Flower Essence Society* organized a worldwide network of flower essence practitioners who report case studies, healing phenomena and patterns associated with flower essence therapy. A professional certification program was developed for training practitioners to work at significant levels of soul healing, and to document clinical results. As a result of this extensive research work with practitioners from around the world, the *Flower Essence Society* formulated an in-depth understanding of flower essence therapy as a *process of soul development*. This process reflects an enhanced understanding of the human soul, just as such knowledge has continued to advance in the wider culture of professional psychotherapy. Three primary components of this research are the following:

A Dynamic Model of Flower Essence Healing

This model is described as the *Four R's of Flower Essence Response,* and is outlined in *Flowers That Heal*[12]. FES case research shows that flower essence therapy can offer more than a palliative or short term healing response. Flower essence healing evokes human potential and involves soul process. Like the plant's movement in metamorphic stages from seed, to leaf, to flower to fruit, the human soul changes in gradual levels of manifestation. All of these stages of development can be stimulated by skillful flower essence therapy.

These four basic levels of response include: initial emotional and/or physical **relief or relaxation**; mental **recognition and realization** of previously

Like the plant's movement in metamorphic stages from seed, to leaf, to flower to fruit, the human soul changes in gradual levels of manifestation. All of these stages of development can be stimulated by skillful flower essence therapy.

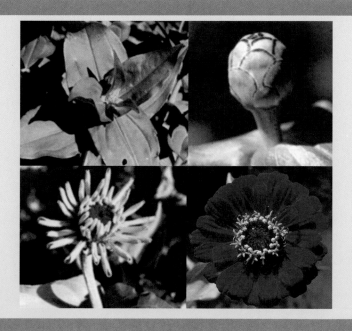

Opening of a Zinnia blossom

hidden aspects of consciousness or behavior; **reaction or resistance** to the flower essence — called the healing crisis — which prompts the "shadow" aspects of the personality to **reconcile conflicting or repressed aspects of behavior** at a deeper point of awareness; and finally **re-constellation and renewal,** so that change is anchored at a profound level, and able to actuate entirely new aspects of human potential. Unless flower essence practitioners are trained to guide the soul in the full possibilities of flower essence use, cases may be concluded prematurely at stage one and sometimes stage two of the therapy.

Meta-Flora Levels of Soul Identity

Extensive research documented by the ***Flower Essence Society*** illustrates eight primary areas of healing addressed by flower essence therapy. These arenas of therapy encompass a multi-level "map" of the human soul. Skillful recognition and appraisal of this wider soul identity is the basis for in-depth training of practitioners in the ***Flower Essence Society.***

Referred to as the ***Meta-Flora Approach to the Human Soul***[13] these levels include:

1) the basic emotional repertoire and belief system inherited from the individual's family and culture at birth;
2) the soul's relationship to bodily identity and capacity for physical presence and vitality in the world;
3) the learning potential of the mind and alchemical capacities of the human soul for discovery and transformation;
4) the ability of the individual to manifest talent and purpose in the world through work and social service;
5) the inner sensitivity and unique creative expression of the soul as manifested in relationships, artistic pursuits and psychic awareness;
6) the ability of the human soul to encounter karma, suffering and death, including the capacity to make amends and to forgive;
7) the core spiritual identity of the soul and its receptivity for transcendent experience;
8) profound awareness for the "Gift of Life on Earth," including the ability to see one's own individual identity actively united with the larger "World Soul."

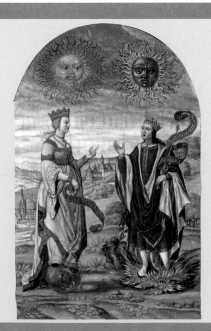

The King Greets the Queen, From Salomon Trismosin, Splendor Solis, 1582

God turns you from one feeling to another and teaches by means of opposites so that you will have two wings to fly, not one. — Rumi

The paradox of life and death returns in a new form at each spiral of growth. If we accept this, we are not torn apart by opposites. — Marion Woodman

The final encompassing level includes aspects of all seven prior stages of development, culminating in a profound reverence within the human soul for life on Earth. This eighth stage was the spiritual goal of all true alchemical work: recognizing that human evolution is inextricably interwoven with the evolution of the living being of Earth (*World Soul* or *Anima Mundi*). From this perspective, we can appreciate that flower essence therapy is a modern re-awakening of alchemical healing, establishing a pathway by which the human soul can live in conscious reciprocity with the soul qualities emanating from Creation.

These **Meta-Flora** levels are not separate phenomena, but dynamic, inter-weaving aspects, like the petals of a flower that form the whole blossom. The task of the competent flower essence practitioner goes beyond *fixing* an immediate problem. The real goal is to awaken and guide the human soul to its own wholeness and integrity. As already well-demonstrated in the field of psychotherapy, there are many sub-personalities or archetypal aspects of the personality that need to come into balance and relationship with each other to form the true *Spiritual Self.* This method of healing through flower essence therapy involves an in-depth approach that differs markedly from the

brief symptom-remedy modality that is more characteristic of medical remediation. *To work proficiently in this new field of therapy, a different paradigm of healing, with an encompassing view of the human being as a bearer of soul consciousness is required.*

The Union of Opposites as the Primary Path of Alchemical Healing

An underlying phenomena in all flower essence therapy involves the concept of alchemical transformation. Alchemy is an ancient art and science, largely misunderstood in our modern era. It entails our relationship to the world of Nature and how the hidden qualities of substances found in Nature can be brought into manifestation through human endeavor. But, it also includes the converse relationship: how the qualities of substances found in Nature likewise affect the interior consciousness of the human being. In its essence, alchemy involves a dynamic and conscious dialogue between the human soul and the soul of Nature. It is this relationship which forms the very foundation of flower essence therapy.

Dr. Bach was a student of alchemy through his membership in the Masonic Lodge. Furthermore, he credits the great alchemist **Paracelsus**[14]

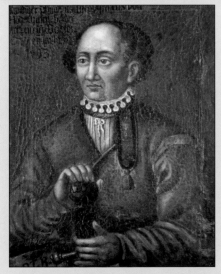

Paracelsus

Just as the flowers grow from the earth, so does the remedy grow in the hands of the physician. ... The remedy is nothing but a seed which you must develop into that which it is destined to be.

Paracelsus

(1493–1541) as one of his noteworthy teachers. Nevertheless, a full exposition of alchemical principles is not presented in Dr. Bach's written work on flower essence therapy. Dr. Bach began his career as an allopathic medical doctor, then left this traditional form of medicine to work as a homeopathic doctor. Dr. Bach considered flower essence therapy to be a distinct departure from homeopathy, but his untimely death prevented him from fully investigating all of its essential differences and distinguishing qualities.

Had he been able to further delineate the new paradigm he was establishing, and analyze his case work for a longer period of time, it is possible that Dr. Bach would have realized its kinship with alchemical principles of healing.

Allopathic medicine cures by prescribing an opposing remedy to the presenting symptom. For instance, an anti-inflammatory drug like aspirin or its herbal counterpart, Willow bark, reduces inflammation, thereby alleviating the external symptom. Homeopathy works by a contrasting principle of similars, or "like cures like," using a remedy that matches the symptom in order to stimulate the body's own healing response. For example, onion (*Allium cepa*) produces tears and nasal discharge and is a typical homeopathic rem-

edy for cold symptoms. Thus allopathic medicine is regarded as a system of diagnosis and cure according to the "law of contraries," while homeopathy works according to the "law of similars."

In his 1931 address, *Ye Suffer from Yourselves*,[15] Dr. Bach urged us to think beyond the work of his renowned teacher, **Samuel Hahnemann**[16] (1755-1843), the founder of homeopathy. He said that we do *not* need remedies based upon the principle of "like cures like" because disease itself matches the inner soul condition, and is a "direct result of wrong thinking and wrong doing." Dr. Bach stated that we need "no longer fight disease with disease ... but bring down the opposing virtue that will eliminate the fault." He went on to claim that "Like may strengthen like, like may repel like, but in the true healing sense like cannot cure like." In his essay published in *Homeopathic World*, **Some Fundamental Considerations of Disease and Cure**[17], Dr. Bach wrote that, "The perfect method is not so much to repel the adverse influence, as to draw in the opposing virtue; and by means of this virtue flood out the fault. This is the law of opposites, of positive and negative."

But did Dr. Bach really introduce a new law of opposites? Are flower essences a novel version of

The genius of Hahnemann realising the nature and reason of disease, used like remedies, which, by temporarily intensifying the illness, hastened its end. He used like poisons to repel the poisons from the body. But having contemplated where his genius left us, let us advance a step further forward, and we shall see that there is even a new and better way.

Edward Bach , "Some Fundamental Considerations of Disease & Cure"

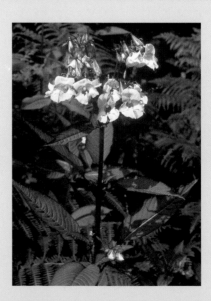

Impatiens:

First prepared by Dr. Bach as a homeopathic remedy in 1928, and then as a flower essence in 1930

allopathic medicine, this time working on the level of the soul, rather than the body? Just as we use an allopathic decongestant to relieve a stuffy head, do we treat the symptom of fear with an antidote like Mimulus that creates calm? Do the flower remedies, "flood our natures with the particular virtue we need, and wash out from us the fault that is causing harm," as Dr. Bach described in *Ye Suffer from Yourselves*? This description bypasses the complexity of the alchemical processes involved in true soul healing, documented and studied with great care by many psychotherapists, but especially Dr. Carl Jung. According to Jung, it is not so much that we rid ourselves of a negative quality, as that we learn to listen to and integrate its healing message. Encountering unconscious or "shadow" aspects of the Self, results in a creative process that calls forth healing archetypes or virtues within the soul.

This truth is borne out in our careful study of flower essence case phenomena. A remedy like Mimulus for example, does not simply create calm. If this were the case, it would act exactly like an allopathic, pharmaceutical tranquilizer that automatically cancels out anxiety without any conscious participation or response from the individual. But a very different process happens when one takes Mimulus. This flower essence helps the indi-

vidual become *aware of fear*, and rouse the necessary *inner forces of courage* to meet the fear. A dynamic dialogue between fear and courage is stimulated, and the soul develops the inner resources to encounter the fear. In studying this phenomena carefully, we can see that there appear to be both allopathic and homeopathic factors in the flower essence method of healing.

Yet, we cannot say that flower essence healing belongs exclusively to *either* category. A third new category of healing is introduced through flower essence therapy that has its roots in the alchemical knowledge of polarities. When opposites come together they are reconciled by a third force, which does not merely replace the two forces, but brings dynamic resolution and balance to them. Thus we can say that flower essence therapy belongs to an entirely new class of healing, which we can call the **Alchemical Union of Opposites.**[18]

As Dr. Jung established, alchemical healing belongs especially to the realm of the human soul, for it is the soul which already, by its very existence, dynamically interacts with the two most fundamental polarities of body and spirit. The very purpose of the human soul is alchemical: it must learn to build a bridge between opposites. This means also that we must formulate a distinct

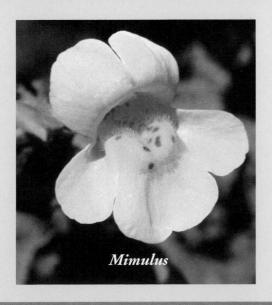

Mimulus

A remedy like Mimulus for example, does not simply create calm. ... This flower essence helps the individual become aware of fear, and rouse the necessary inner forces of courage to meet the fear.

healing paradigm that differs from that of bodily medicine. Such an understanding is vital in the successful execution of flower essence therapy. Without this perspective, we will relegate flower essence therapy to the realm of allopathic medical healing and externally-oriented symptom-remedy resolution, failing to utilize the deepest healing potential of flower essences for the soul-developmental process.

The early flower essence casework of Dr. Bach demonstrates that the understanding of these major healing principles outlined above had not been completely worked through at that time. For example, a typical case presented by Dr. Bach in a 1933 homeopathic journal[19] describes an 18-year old girl who had recurring cysts. She was a gentle, introverted soul who daydreamed, thus Clematis was selected and administered three times a day for one week. During this time period, the cysts were absorbed. The remedy was maintained for three more months, and because there was no recurrence of the cysts, the case was deemed successful and concluded. This case emphasizes the use of a flower essence for the Stage One level of response, providing palliative relief from physical symptoms. The case does not explore the inner dynamic within the young girl's soul, and this factor was evidently not deemed important enough to discuss in the case report. Thus, the success of the case was evaluated according to the resolution of the presenting physical symptom.

This case, like most of those presented in the work of Dr. Bach and his colleagues, Phillip Chancellor[20] and Nora Weeks, are of relatively short duration. We do not follow the longitudinal development of the individual, and the fuller aspects of identity and human potential that can be fostered in a comprehensive *Meta-Flora Approach to the Human Soul*. Such an understanding is only possible through the further application of the laws and principles governing psychotherapeutic alchemical healing, and the collection and analysis of many more cases than were possible to obtain in the short seven years of Dr. Bach's ground-breaking research.

Pioneering a Living Science of Nature

Another significant area of research addressed by the *Flower Essence Society* during the last two decades, involves the scientific study of plants. Even though we may clearly note the effectiveness of flower essences in clinical cases, how do we account for the radically different way Dr. Bach developed plant essences, so that they are correlated with the condition of the soul itself? The work

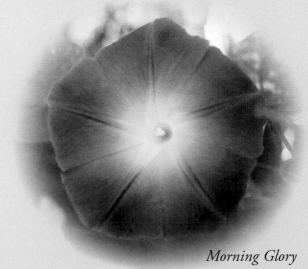

A morning glory at my window satisfies me more than the metaphysics of books.   Walt Whitman

Morning Glory

of Dr. Bach runs counter to medical science and even to traditional medical herbalism. For centuries, plant science has been directed toward diagnosis and alleviation of physical symptoms, correlated with precise chemical constituents in plants. Modern medical science emphasizes more detailed biochemical analysis and the development of synthetic compounds, originally derived from plants, but now artificially formulated in pharmaceutical laboratories.

When we delve deeper into the spiritual roots of all cultures, we find that many plants were associated with emotional and spiritual states of consciousness. Yet Dr. Bach's contribution is far more than a revival of ancient shamanic plant wisdom or the ritualistic use of plants. His training as a medical doctor enabled him to understand human suffering and plants in a manner that speaks to the modern condition of consciousness. Each plant is correlated with a precise state of soul-consciousness in a manner that had never before been achieved, either in modern medical science or in ancient plant wisdom.

Here again, Dr. Bach was truly a pioneer. But although he entered new territory in a successful and convincing manner, the detailed map of the terrain was not available. Writing in *The Medical Discoveries of Dr. Edward Bach*[21], his colleague, Nora Weeks, described Bach as a keen sensitive, able to "feel" the energies of plants as he sat with them, or tasted their blossoms. We also know that Dr. Bach spent countless hours walking in Nature and observing plants carefully. Weeks reported that Bach "spent the day examining a great variety of plants, noting where they grew, what soil they chose to grow upon, the colour, shape and number of their petals, whether they spread by tuber, root or seed. ... " He devoted hours studying "the habits and characteristics of each flower, plant and tree." Dr. Bach urged Weeks to recognize each of the remedy plants at every stage of its growth. Julian Barnard, the world's foremost scholar and practitioner of Dr. Bach's work, has written a noteworthy new book, *Bach Flower Remedies: Form & Function,*[22] shedding light on how we can understand Bach's plant research. Barnard weaves together detailed plant observations, based upon Bach's scant commentary, and his own perceptive insights. Barnard's work is an outstanding contribution by an author who has spent many hours in the field in devoted contemplation of Bach's plants.

While Dr. Bach's original writings contain only cursory references to the descriptions and signatures of the plants themselves, Dr. Bach's selection

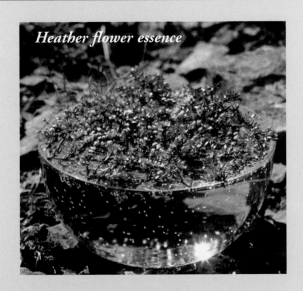

Heather flower essence

Dr. Bach's contribution is far more than a revival of ancient shamanic plant wisdom or the ritualistic use of plants. His training as a medical doctor enabled him to understand human suffering and plants in a manner that speaks to the modern condition of consciousness. Each plant is correlated with a precise state of soul-consciousness in a manner that had never before been achieved, either in modern medical science or in ancient plant wisdom.

of certain healing plants must be regarded as the work of a trained medical doctor. Spiritual inspiration was surely operative, but if his insights were only subjective or vague psychic impressions, Dr. Bach's work would not have endured and flourished throughout the world. Dr. Bach approached a new vista, but did not have time in his short life of fifty years to outline a systematic method for understanding his ground-breaking work with plant qualities.

For this reason, we have continued to build on the foundation given to us by Dr. Bach. We have sought to develop a systematic method of study that bridges the polarity of science and spirituality. In this quest, we have been guided by the studies of the German naturalist and poet, **Johann Goethe**[23] (1749-1832). Goethe's work is further developed in the Anthroposophic spiritual science of **Rudolf Steiner**[24] (1861-1925), and in Biodynamic Agriculture and Anthroposophic Medicine, which developed out of Steiner's research. Steiner's central teaching, modeled upon Goethean science, is that we learn to behold all substances and phenomena in Nature from the perspective of human imagination, inspiration and intuition; yet at the same time apply logical thinking, clarity of consciousness and awake sense-per-

ception to our investigations. For an extended discussion of the historical, cultural and scientific context for the FES plant studies, please see the following article, *The Living Science of Nature,* starting on page 32.

The **Flower Essence Society** has applied and extended many of these methods of investigation in learning to understand the qualities of the original plants indicated by Dr. Bach and many other important new remedies. FES field studies comprise a multi-dimensional view of the plant, which is characterized as **Twelve Windows of Plant Perception.**[25] Such an approach includes the study of form and gesture of the plant; its orientation in space; botanical plant family affiliation; time cycles which rule the growth of the plant; environmental relationships; the precise signatures of one or more of the four elements which influence the plant; the relationship of the plant to the other kingdoms of Nature; the significance of color as a distinct quality in the plant signature; the over-all sensory experience of the plant including taste, fragrance or touch; chemical or nutritional components of the plant; known medicinal and herbal uses; and relevant folk wisdom, mythology and lore.

These studies differ from conventional analytical science in that many diverse qualities of the

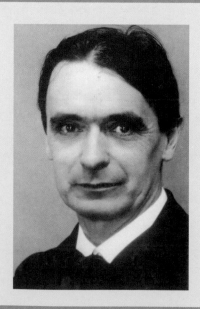

The plant-world is the mirror of human conscience in external nature. Nothing more poetical can be imagined than the thought of this voice of conscience coming forth from some point within us and being distributed over the myriad forms of the blossoming plants which speak to the soul, during the season of the year, in the most manifold ways. The plant-world reveals itself as the wide-spread mirror of conscience if we know how to look at it aright.

Rudolf Steiner, Harmony of the Creative Word

plant, as well as physical factors, are considered. The aim is to build a cohesive picture of the plant that includes various dimensions of knowing. Through these efforts a holistic view of the plant emerges, helping to determine its ability to heal soul states of consciousness. While these investigations are a clear departure from materialistic science, they are also very distinct from disembodied psychic approaches derived from trance channeling, or subjective impressions that are not grounded in physical observation or objective perception. These initial plant studies are further refined and corroborated through practitioner reports and related clinical phenomena, until a cohesive, yet living picture of each flower remedy is achieved.

In order to provide a very brief illustration of this approach to plant study, we can compare and contrast several well-known flower essences in the Sunflower (Asteraceae or Compositae) and Rose (Rosaceae) botanical plant families. Although there are numerous avenues for building a complete picture of plant properties and qualities, the main focus for the purpose of this limited essay will be on basic botanical distinctions. These rudimentary plant sketches can offer insight into several of Dr. Bach's original remedies and consideration of additional plant essences that expand these healing themes.

Asteraceae (Compositae) Plant Family

The Asteraceae botanical plant family is also known as the "Composite" or "Sunflower" Family. Plants in this family comprise a vast spectrum, particularly notable for the geometric precision and detailed intricacy of the flowers. The complex flower head generally contains a central core of disk or tubular florets surrounded by petal-like ray or strap florets, hence the name "composite." From a botanical point of view, the "one" flower we see is actually composed of many single flowers brought together — in effect a microcosmic meadow of hundreds of tiny flowers radiates from each flower head!

The Composite Family of plants is regarded as a more recent, and more advanced, expression of evolution within plant life. The regenerative forces of the plant are richly concentrated in their seed heads, with the potential for enormous genetic diversity, in contrast to simple vegetative replication of the same genetic material through rhizomous roots, runners or bulbs. Thus, the flowers of the composite plants impress us with a kind of

Every natural fact is a symbol of some spiritual fact ... the world is emblematic. The laws of moral nature answer to those of matter as face to face in a glass.

Ralph Waldo Emerson

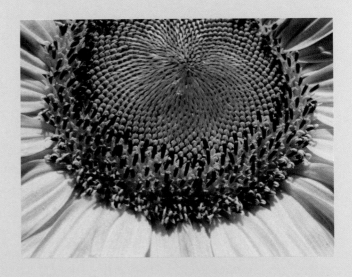

Sunflower Family flowers are actually a composite of many disk and ray florets: a miniature meadow on a stalk!

"wakefulness" and clear individuality, replete with distinctively detailed forms and vivid structures.

Viewed from another perspective, the various members of the "sunflower" family evoke a picture of the sun itself, with its awake "eye" of light. (The daisy — or "day's eye" — is another name for this plant family.) Like the rays of the composite flowers, the various planets find their harmonic "center" through cyclic rotations around the eye of the sun. The alchemical dictum, "as above, so below," guides us to see that this same sun force also exists as a core element of consciousness within each individual human soul. The "I" or ego anchors the idea of "self" within the human soul by integrating and harmonizing its various archetypes and sub-personalities into one cohesive wholeness, not unlike the composite flower with its many separate flowers that form one luminous totality.

Thus, we can appreciate the capacity of the composite flowers to strengthen various aspects of self-identity. On the physical level, they are powerful allies for the immune system. On the soul level, they enhance clarity of consciousness and the capacity for integration and balance of the many aspects of the self-identity, mediated by a core spiritual awareness.

The towering, bright-yellow **Sunflower** (*Helianthus annuus*) blooms in the full glory of the warm summer. Its homage to the sun is striking, for it literally turns its head throughout the course of the sun's daily cycle, to stay in alignment with the sun's rays. The sunflower forms a large head that becomes too heavy for the structure of the plant to support, and must eventually surrender itself to earth's gravity. We see in the gesture of this plant, a striking regal, solar quality, but also a quality of surrender and homage to the earth. The Sunflower essence is used to address the masculine, solar aspect of the soul in both men and women, balancing the polarities of self-aggrandizement and self-effacement with the goal of developing healthy ego expression.

Native to American prairies and open spaces, **Echinacea** (*Echinacea purpurea*) is a woody perennial, growing from a strong root, with an impressive, firm stem. The flower head is filled with bristly, dark tubular florets forming a bulging cone, surrounded by bright magenta ray florets. In the Echinacea plant, one finds a synthesis of unyielding vigor of physical form, with the etheric aliveness in its bright fiery core and vibrant magenta blossoms radiating in the brilliant light of the high summer sun. As we study the form and

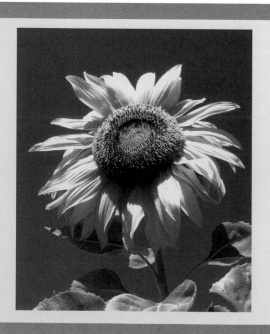

We see in the gesture of the Sunflower, a striking regal, solar quality, but also a quality of surrender and homage to the earth.

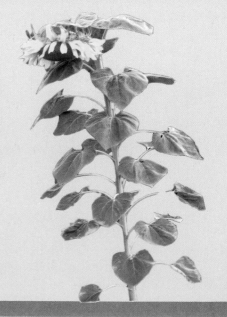

gesture of the Echinacea, it is apparent why it is widely recognized as an immune system remedy, used to increase resistance to influenza and other infectious diseases. Even holding or standing next to the plant, one feels a surge of strengthening forces that instill firmness and confidence. The flower essence of Echinacea is used for many challenges to the "immunity" of the Soul. The anonymity of modern civilization, along with countless other mechanizing and alienating forces such as crime, violence, and sexual or emotional degradation, can shatter the dignity of the Self. Echinacea flower essence stimulates and awakens genuine Self-consciousness. A lack of essential self-respect erodes the health of the soul, and is a hidden factor in many immune abnormalities in our time.

Cosmos *Cosmos bipinnatus* — Unlike the Sunflower, with its stately and long-lived flowering gesture, the Cosmos grows a bounty of flowers in rapid succession, beginning early in summer and lasting well into autumn. The quality of movement in air is quite pronounced in this plant and can be seen even in the finely divided feathery leaves and flower petals. It makes sense that butterflies are attracted to this plant, flitting about the flowers with ever-changing movements that somehow echo the spirit of the flower. Indeed, the plant

essence of Cosmos helps to quicken the mercurial activity of consciousness in the human soul. The vibrant forces of vitality that we find in the ever-blooming magenta-pink blossoms, benefit the thinking and speech activities of consciousness that may be weighed down and dull, or disorganized and inarticulate. Cosmos seems a fitting name for this flower that reflects the higher logos activity of consciousness in the human soul.

Madia *Madia elegans* — Madia is a native wildflower found in open and dry slopes in the coastal hills, foothills and moderate mountain elevations of California. Linear leaves are arranged alternately along the stem, and both the leaves and stem are hairy and sticky, giving the Madia the common name of "Tarweed." Madia features bright yellow ray florets and yellow tubular (disk) florets. The variety prepared as a flower essence is characterized by ray florets with three-lobed tips and maroon-red spots at the base, appearing as a striking red ring in the center of the flower. The flower forms a living *mandala,* bringing the attention to focus on its center.

Madia begins blooming in June and continues until October, when most of the surrounding foliage has dried up. An unusual characteristic of this composite, is that the flowers open in late

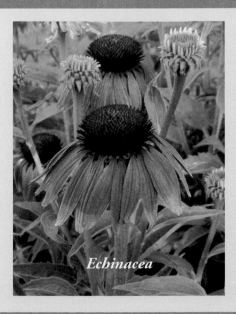

Echinacea

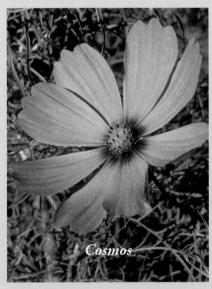

Cosmos

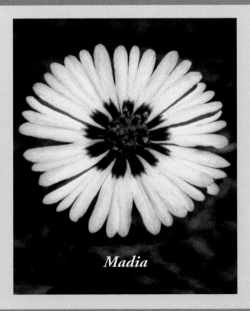

Madia

afternoon and remain open until the following mid-morning. However, during the intense heat of the mid-day sun, the ray flowers curl inward and the flower is nearly invisible.

The remarkable ability of Madia to remain blooming over a long period, and to pull inward during the time of day when the forces of light and heat are most expansive, is correlated with a condition in the human soul involving distraction, excessive sanguinity and diffuse mental forces. The red ring of color at the center of this flower suggests a vital, "inwardizing" quality of consciousness, and indeed, the Madia flower essence enhances the capacity to retain focus and centered awareness, or "self-consciousness."

Dandelion *Taraxacum officinale* — The yellow Dandelion bursts forth, exalting in the bright glory of spring's first sunny days. Named for the Old French *dent-de-lion*, or "tooth of the lion," because of its jagged tooth-like leaves and flowers, Dandelion displays impressive energetic qualities. Its long tap root extends deeply into the ground, and in early spring the sturdy green stem shoots quickly forward, erupting with "lion-toothed" leaves. The flowers of the "dandy lion" roar with solar fire, then quickly become airy balls of crystal-fine seed released with exuberant abandon in the wind. It is interesting to note that Dandelion belongs to a tribe within the Sunflower family that are exclusively "ray" flowers, without any center. It does seem that Dandelion is a pronounced plant "extrovert," with its rapid, impulsive growth and seemingly ubiquitous presence that has earned it the unwarranted status of "weed." The essence of this flower is most beneficial for soul conditions of strong intensity and drive, leading to over-exertion and muscular tension. Such individuals exploit the life forces, especially those related to the organ of the liver. They need to develop an interior "center" of consciousness that balances the overly-active will (or doing) aspect of soul, so that mindfulness gives form and substance to passionate activity.

Chicory *Cichorium intybus* — Chicory has delicate, paper-thin, blue flowers that bloom in the earliest part of the day. The flowers on a single plant are multitudinous, yet each one lasts for only a few hours until the ephemeral petals seem to evaporate into the blue of the late morning sky. Like the Dandelion, there are no central disk flowers on this plant, only the fragile, ever-waning ray flowers. Yet there are striking differences as well as similarities. Unlike the bright yellow, extroverted activity of the Dandelion, the delicate blue flowers of the Chicory point to a different quality of soul

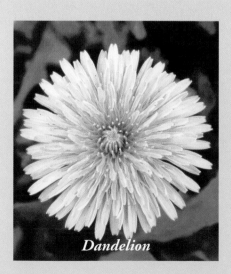
Dandelion

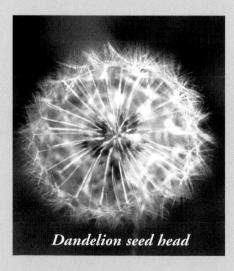
Dandelion seed head

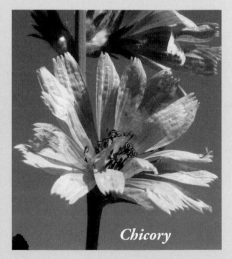
Chicory

experience. As Dr. Bach indicated, Chicory is for a type of emotional grasping that can become manipulative and "self-centered," in the negative sense of the word. Such individuals do not have an authentic "core" self that contains and harmonizes soul experience, providing objective consciousness. The clinging, overly needy and congested state of the soul is helped by this plant which blooms so freely, constantly giving over its substance to the spiritual world. When the higher witness of the Self-identity replaces the narrow emotions of the lower personality, love flows more freely, and in the words of Dr. Bach, "we can open up both our arms and bless all around."[26]

The low-growing, continually-blooming **Calendula** (*Calendula officinalis*), also known as Mary's Gold, imparts a unique feminine quality of soul consciousness in this "solar" plant family. Most Composite Family plants ray out like stars, but the Calendula's inflorescence forms a chalice of soft, fragrant, gently-curving flowers exuding a warm, golden color and powerful etheric vitality. Thus this plant is called "Mary's Gold" because it forms such an exquisite container for holding the sun's warmth, with herbal properties that are softening and soothing for the skin. The Calendula helps the egocentric individual who needs to learn how to express social warmth, and to hold the ego presence of others with sensitive and compassionate attention. Calendula represents a unique quality within this family of plants that heal various kinds of self-consciousness: this flower essence addresses the feminine capacity to become receptive to the "I-Self" of another, as part of one's own fuller identity.

Rosaceae Plant Family

The Rose family (Rosaceae) of plants has exceptionally integrated qualities of strength and beauty. In general, its members have a strong drive for incarnation and are rooted in the rich substance of earth. In contrast to the Asteraceae family with strong reproductive qualities in the seed "heads," roses regenerate with their "feet," and typically gain vitality when cut back or pruned. Yet, in spite of tenacious and resilient roots, penetrating thorns and woody bark, the blossoms from the Rose Family plants have redolent, ethereal fragrances which are neither overwhelmingly intoxicating nor acutely pungent, and fruits that are tart or mildly sweet. No members of this family are poisonous, and most yield highly nutritional foods or salutary medicines.

The ability of the Rose Family to bring spiritual forces into fruitful manifestation on earth, is a

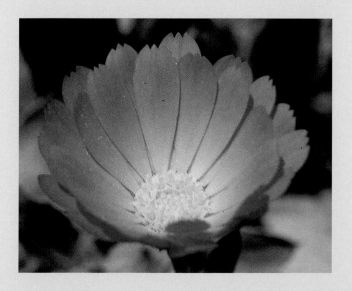

Calendula's inflorescence forms a chalice of soft, fragrant, gently-curving flowers exuding a warm, golden color and powerful etheric vitality.

picture for the human soul of how love becomes an active force of willing, serving and giving. Thus the fruits and medicinal tonics made from the Rose Family revitalize and cleanse the blood, energize the metabolism, tone digestive processes and nourish reproductive capacities.

The geometric form which rules the roses is the five-pointed star. In history, mythology and folk custom, the rose is associated with human love, and especially with the planet, Venus. This cosmic truth is reflected in the heavens, where the planet Venus inscribes a five-pointed star in her conjunctions with the Sun, as viewed from the earth. The rose is enchantingly beautiful, but it also has its fierce side of prickly thorns and resolute roots. As soul medicines, the Rose Family plants anchor and sustain cosmic ideals within the human body and the body of the earth. In this sense, the tender Venusian mysteries of love are interwoven with the polar opposite forces of fiery Mars, helping human ideals manifest through deeds on earth.

In the human body, the dynamic expression of the five-pointed star is formed by the "doing" part of ourselves: our feet and hands actively streaming between heaven and earth. Two star forms are created — the external star, as well as an ethereal center in the heart region. This "inner star," or "breastplate," is shaped like a pentagon. The Rose Family teaches us about love as an active expression of the heart. When the "willing" part of the human soul can illumine its "star" of cosmic ideals, our heart center blossoms on earth as does a rose.

Wild Rose (*Rosa canina*) (also known as Dog Rose, the one prepared by Dr. Bach) and **California Wild Rose** (*Rosa californica*) are closely related plants that are consummate representatives of the Rose Family. As such, they are foundational flower essences that are widely used for the most basic issues of love and idealism within the human soul. Growing freely as rambling shrubs at the edges of woodlands and in other marginal areas, wild roses thrive in poor soils, with abundant root systems that break ground with fresh growth whenever the plant dies back, or is grazed by animals. The flowers are subtle pink with lusciously delicate fragrance, while the rose hips (fruits) are bright red.

A significant feature of the wild roses are their thorns. If we carefully observe the growth pattern of roses, we can discover that the thorns are nodal points that would have produced additional leaves and branches much earlier in the development process. The beauty that we see in the rose flower is literally produced through a trial of thorns. The

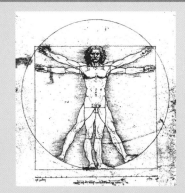 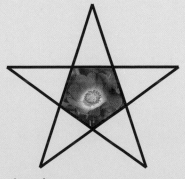 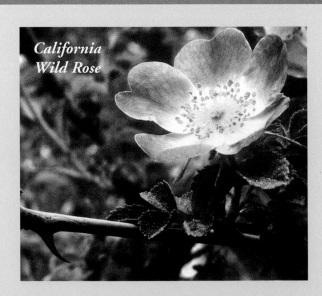

California Wild Rose

In the human body, the dynamic expression of the five-pointed star is formed by the "doing" part of ourselves: our feet and hands actively streaming between heaven and earth.

physical power of the plant has become focused and well-contained, learning how to endure and embrace the forces of the earth. Through this process of sublimation, the rose produces its ethereal five-pointed star blossom.

With this picture in mind, we can see how the flower essences of California Wild Rose and English Wild Rose heal many forms of alienation and apathy in the soul. These essences help individuals who shun full incarnation into physical life on earth, especially the pain or "thorns" of earthly striving. The soul needs to discover that only through earthly challenges, can love become a radiant force within the soul. The California Wild Rose brings enthusiasm and joy for life, working particularly on the soul's loss of ideals and commitment, resulting in disinterest, boredom, depression, cynicism, and, in extreme instances, suicidal tendencies. Dr. Bach's Wild Rose addresses conditions which manifest particularly through the body, such as the inability to recover from illness and related states of malaise and impassivity about one's physical condition.

Blackberry *Rubus ursinus* — Anyone who has encountered a brier patch of blackberry brambles knows that they are a much more intense version of the wild rose. The flowers of the blackberry are white, and similar in form to the wild rose, but its fruits are dark and contracted, with a piquant sweetness. The intense concentration of force which the dark-fruited blackberry harbors is strikingly evident in its dense tangle of thorns, which are stronger, thicker and broader than typical roses. Blackberry shrubs have amazing regenerative abilities, spreading vigorously and quickly with horizontal runners. As any gardener who has ever tried to remove blackberries knows, the smallest bit of root left in the earth will immediately break ground with fresh new growth forces.

Within the spectrum of Rose Family plants, blackberry can be considered as having the strongest earthy forces, growing on the horizon of the earth in parallel streams of energy, extending its rampageous "limbs" with great zest, and covering considerable space in a very short amount of time. These qualities make Blackberry flower essence an excellent remedy for those who are unable to radiate will forces through their limbs. Although there may be many good intentions and ideals, practical manifestation is much more difficult. Such individuals live more readily in spiritual and mental spheres and can have a sluggish metabolism. Blackberry flower essence ignites the will, revitalizes the blood and instills a more dynamic

Within the Rose Family plants, Blackberry can be considered as having the strongest earthy forces ... extending its rampageous "limbs" with great zest, and covering considerable space in a very short amount of time.

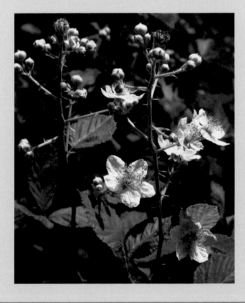
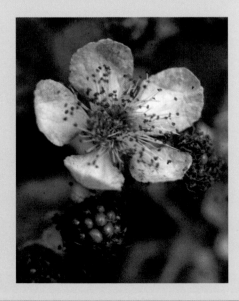

relationship with the physical body and earthly life.

Quince *Chaenomeles speciosa* — To behold the blossoming Quince in early spring can stir the most hardened soul. Flowering quite early when winter still threatens, one is struck by exquisitely silky, deep-pink blossoms sitting atop the dark, thorn-studded branches of the Quince. In some cases, the blossoms appear entirely alone, and in other instances, some beginning leaf growth accompanies the flowers. The fruit of the Quince is markedly astringent, and it is significant to note that its seeds are an effective medical treatment for hay fever. Allergic reactions like hay fever develop when the air element within the human soul is hypersensitive and cannot contract sufficiently to accommodate the etheric-physical body. As with the other Rose Family plants, we see within the Quince, a particular way in which the soul is guided to incarnation on earth.

The flower essence of the Quince treats the hypersensitivity of the soul in a unique manner. It is particularly indicated for those who have enormous capacities for love but do not know how to balance their heart forces with inner conviction and soul strength. Quince flower essence is also beneficial for those whose lifestyle requires keen balance

of seemingly opposite soul forces — such as parents or teachers who must learn to be both firm and nurturing with the children under their care.

Cherry Plum *Prunus cerasifera* — Like the Quince, Cherry Plum (one of Dr. Bach's remedies) retains its germinal structure throughout winter, sending forth blossoms directly from dark brown wood when winter wanes and the first sunlit days of spring emerge. The white flowers have a soft, radiant purity, impressing the soul with harmonious calm and peace. The Cherry Plum is a transitional plant in the Rose Family spectrum, it is not quite a shrub, and yet can only be considered a very small tree. The Cherry Plum does not possess the abundant thorns of the wild roses, but has some thorns, unlike more developed orchard fruit trees such as apple, pear or peach, that are entirely thornless.

The Cherry Plum flower essence has qualities which are complementary to the Quince. Whereas the Quince personality has pronounced sensitivity that does not contain enough firmness and strength, the Cherry Plum type holds on too tightly, suffering from extreme mental and physical rigidity. Intense fear of losing control leads to excessive tension in the body and many forms of apprehension and dread. The flower essence of

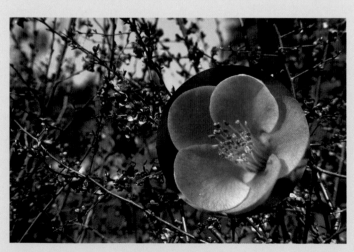

Quince

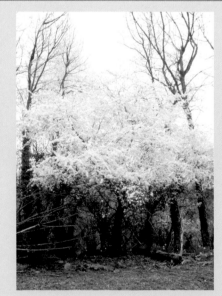

Cherry Plum

Cherry Plum helps the soul to learn trust and surrender by establishing *concordance* — literally meaning to live within the harmonic sphere of the heart or *core* of the Self. Of all Rose Family plants, one is struck by the sheer transcendence of the blossoming Cherry Plum, with clouds of white flowers that have surrendered their essence in the most pure manner to the cosmos. Thus, Cherry Plum is one of the important five flowers in the famous emergency combination of Dr. Bach, used to address extreme states of distress and pain, by easing excessive contraction and tension.

Crab Apple *Malus sylvestris* — Domestic apple trees are more lush and of greater physical stature than the Crab Apple, yet this species is one of the original wild apples from which domestic varieties have emerged. It is a small tree that is scrubby in appearance with its dark striated bark and gnarled trunk. There is a splendid quality in the very wildness of the Crab Apple, with its ardent physical embrace of the earth, blooming in spring with voluptuous masses of fragrant white flowers blushed with pink contours, and culminating in autumn with compact golden fruits.

The apple has a strong mythological significance in human culture. In Celtic lore, *Avalon* literally means the *Isle of Apples*, where the goddesses of healing and immortality dwell. In Greek and Roman mythology, the apple is regarded as the fruit of Venus, the goddess of love. The book of Genesis describes the Tree of Life which bears fruit and grows in Paradise, and it is typically depicted as an apple tree. However, when the apple is eaten, the human soul can no longer live in the ethereal dimension of Paradise, but must find its way into the earthly realm and physical incarnation.

Crab Apple represents another variation upon the theme of earthly love and incarnation, which the Rose Family represents so evocatively. The flower essence is indicated for those who feel the imperfection of bodily existence and long for the paradisiacal unity of pre-earthly consciousness. The slightest blemish, physical malfunction or illness is difficult to accept or transform, and receives exaggerated focus and hypercritical attention. Another application of the Crab Apple flower essence is for those who may have "fallen" too much into the density of physical existence; such individuals need strong cleansing and revitalizing forces in the metabolism, especially digestion, elimination or sexual reproduction. In either instance, the Crab Apple helps the soul integrate cosmic and physical identities, so that the body and soul may work with greater harmony and equanimity on earth.

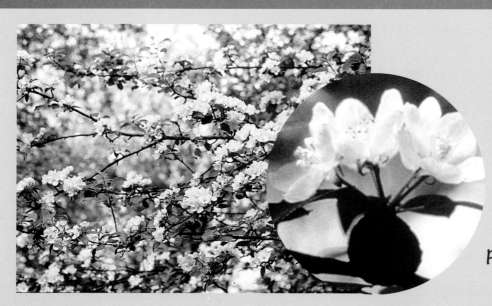

Crab Apple flower essence is indicated for those who feel the imperfection of bodily existence and long for the paradisiacal unity of pre-earthly consciousness.

Agrimony *Agrimonia eupatoria* — In contrast to the thorny bushes or fruiting trees of the Rose Family, Agrimony represents another variation within the impressive range of this botanical group. It is a herbaceous perennial that thrives in open meadows and woodlands with sunny yellow flowers. Agrimony has a strong vertical orientation and is appropriately named "church steeples." It grows upwards in a straight line, with pinnate leaves that metamorphose into a densely-clustered floral spike. The aroma and taste of the Agrimony is quite fiery, and reminiscent of cloves. The spine and leaves of the Agrimony are rough and covered with many hairs; one almost expects to find thorns somewhere on the plant. But the thorny feature is not in its typical place—instead, one finds spiny hooks in the receptacles. These bristly burrs hold the golden flowers of the Agrimony and later become tenacious fruits and seeds that readily adhere to clothing or animal fur. Whereas the fierce aspect of most members of the Rose Family is typically observed in the roots, thorns, bark or stem, here we see that the flowering process itself has a thorn-like quality.

The Agrimony personality represents another variation on the theme of balance and equilibrium between cosmic and earthly poles. The Agrimony type attempts to present a harmonious cosmic exterior to the world at the expense of troubling emotions or shadow aspects of the personality that are suppressed. The strong spiritual aspirations of the Agrimony type are represented in the way this plant grows in such straight lines with its flowering "church steeples." Yet, hidden within the cosmic aspirations of the flowering soul are the "burrs" of troubling emotions which must be acknowledged and integrated. This member of the Rose Family teaches us an important lesson about human love — only by encountering what seems lower and filled with thorns or challenges, can the soul grow in true balance between earthly and cosmic poles.

Lady's Mantle *Alchemilla vulgaris* — Lady's Mantle is an exceptional member of the Rose Family that stands at the far end of its diverse spectrum of plant members. This Rosaceae representative is almost all leaf and does not grow vertically but spreads on the surface of the earth, with modest flowers that are golden green. Lady's Mantle has a marvelous ability to attract and hold dew. Sparkling beads of water grace this plant long after moisture has evaporated in the surrounding gardens and meadows. The palmate leaves of the Lady's Mantle are curved, creating a single,

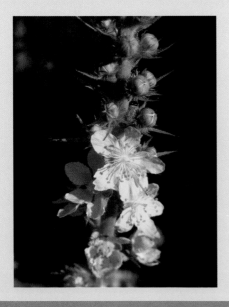

The strong spiritual aspirations of the Agrimony type are represented in the way this plant grows in such straight lines with its flowering "church steeples." Yet, hidden within the cosmic aspirations of the flowering soul are the "burrs" of troubling emotions which must be acknowledged and integrated.

rounded form; they are literally *chalices* which receive the dew of earth and offer it to the heavens.

Alchemists regard dew as a primal healing essence that exudes from the earth when the four elements of earth, air, fire and water are in harmonious balance. From the macrocosmic perspective, the blue-green Earth herself can be viewed as a precious dewdrop floating in cosmic space. Dr. Bach recognized the precious gift of dew formation and originally prepared flower essences by gathering their dew in the early morning. This method was gradually perfected by picking flowers at the peak of their seasonal blossoming in the early morning time of the ascending sun, when dew forces impregnate the earth. The flowers are infused in a crystal bowl (chalice) of local spring water, interweaving the other three elements of earth, air and fire during the medicine-making process.

The "Leaf Chalice" of *Alchemilla* stays in close harmony with the earth, so that even her flower retains the green colour of the earth's etheric sheath. Thus, her other name of "Lady's Mantle" is also fitting, for she literally cloaks the earth with beneficent forces of healing dew. The Lady's Mantle herb is a well known remedy for women, especially benefiting the uterus. For example, it is used to revitalize the reproductive system after birth. The uterus has a strong relationship — both in physiology and form — to the heart, and in many healing systems is regarded as a "second heart" within each woman. The "uterus heart" aligns each woman with the mothering forces within the heart of the Earth itself.

As a flower essence, the Lady's Mantle is indicated for women with a strong history of reproductive trauma, who may bear within their wombs not only their own personal suffering, but also the longing for the Earth herself. It is also helpful for healers, teachers and others who aspire to work from their highest ideals to serve others. Just as the successful gardener needs a "green thumb," the plant healer needs a "green heart." This means that healing involves an innate recognition that the Earth is a living being, and that the chalice of one's own heart be able to emanate soul qualities within Nature.

As a whole, the Rose Family teaches us how to develop our heart forces, so that human love mediates between Heaven and Earth. Within this theme, the Lady's Mantle plays a most exceptional role, helping to align the human heart with the heart of the living Earth. It is most fitting that she is called *Alchemilla* for her essence represents the goal of all genuine alchemical healing, especially flower essence therapy.

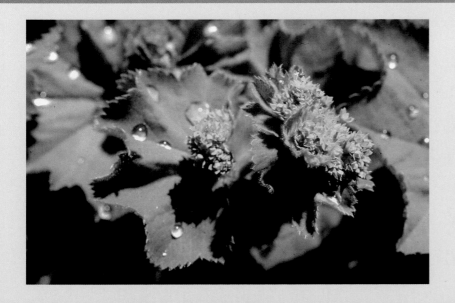

Lady's Mantle (Alchemilla) has an extraordinary ability to collect and hold dew. Its palmate leaves are curved, creating a single rounded form; they are literally chalices which receive the dew of earth and offer it to the heavens.

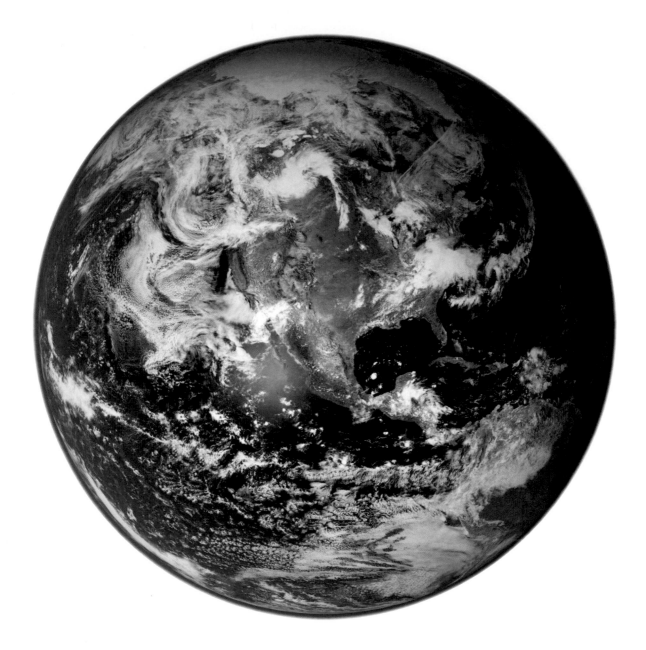

When we contemplate the whole globe as one great dewdrop, striped and dotted with continents and islands, flying through space with other stars — all singing and shining together as one, the whole universe appears as an infinite storm of beauty.

— John Muir, *The Story of My Boyhood and Youth*

End Notes

1. Weeks, Nora, *The Medial Discoveries of Edward Bach, Physician,* C.W. Daniel, Co, Ltd, Saffron Walden, Essex, England, 1940. This is the primary biographical reference for Dr. Bach, and is the source for the basic outline of his life as presented in this article. The quotation from Nora Weeks on page 9 is taken from this book.

2. Described in Bach, Edward, "Some New Remedies and New Uses," p. 6, *Homoeopathic World,* February, 1930 and "Some Fundamental Considerations of Disease & Cure," p. 13, *Homeopathic World,* December, 1930. Published in Barnard, Julian, *Collected Writings of Edward Bach,* Ashgrove Press, London, 1999.

3. Described in Bach, Edward, "Some Fundamental Considerations of Disease & Cure," p. 15, *Homeopathic World,* December, 1930.

4. Described in Bach, Edward, "Some New Remedies and New Uses," p. 5, *Homoeopathic World,* February, 1930. Bach used the leaves of this remedy, as this was before he discovered the true flower essence method.

5. See Barnard, Julian, *Collected Writings of Edward Bach,* Ashgrove Press, London, 1999, to see the various stages of Bach's work as expressed in the subsequent editions of *The Twelve Healers.*

6. Bach, Edward, "Some Fundamental Considerations of Disease & Cure," p. 5, *Homeopathic World,* December, 1930. Published in Barnard, Julian, *Collected Writings of Edward Bach,* Ashgrove Press, London, 1999.

7. Selye, Hans "A Syndrome Produced by Diverse Nocuous Agents.*" Nature,* 1936, 138, 32. See also Selye, Hans, *The Stress of Life,* McGraw-Hill, New York, NY, 1956, 1978.

8. See Maslow, Abraham, *Motivation and Personality,* Addison-Wesley, Boston, MA, 1987; Maslow, Abraham, *The Farther Reaches of Personality,* Arkana, New York, 1993; and Maslow, Abraham, *Toward a Psychology of Being,* John Wiley and Sons, Hoboken, NJ, 1998.

9. See Jung, Carl, *Collected Works of C.G. Jung:* Vol 12: *Psychology and Alchemy;* Vol 13: *Alchemical Studies,* Vol 14: *Mysterium Coniunctionis;* University Press, Princeton NJ, 1977, 1983.

10. See Assagioli, Roberto, *Psychosynthesis, A Collection of Basic Writings,* The Synthesis Center; Amherst, MA, 2000.

11. See Frankl, Viktor, *Man's Search for Meaning,* Washington Square Press, New York, 1985.

12. Kaminski, Patricia, *Flowers that Heal,* Gill and Macmillan, Dublin, Ireland, 1998.

13. See *Flowers that Heal* for a summary of the Meta-Flora levels. Further writing on this topic is in preparation.

14. See Paracelsus, *Selected Writings,* Jolande Jacobi, ed., Princeton University Press, Princeton, NJ, 1995.

15. Published in Barnard, Julian, *Collected Writings of Edward Bach,* Ashgrove Press, London, 1999.

16. Hahnemann, Samuel, *Organon der Heilkunst [Organon of Healing],* 1833 (out of print).

17. Published in Barnard, Julian, *Collected Writings of Edward Bach,* Ashgrove Press, London, 1999.

18. See Jung, Carl, *Collected Works of C.G. Jung:* Vol 14: *Mysterium Coniunctionis,* Princeton, University Press, 1977.

19. Bach, Edward, "Twelve Great Remedies," page 85 from *Heal Thyself* (homeopathic journal), 1933, reprinted in Barnard, Julian, *Collected Writings of Edward Bach,* Ashgrove Press, London, 1999.

20. Chancellor, Philip, *Illustrated Handbook of the Bach Flower Remedies,* C.W. Daniel, Co, Ltd., Essex, England, 1977, 1996.

21. Weeks, Nora, *The Medical Discoveries of Edward Bach, Physician,* C.W. Daniel, Co, Ltd., Essex, England, 1940, 1973, 1998.

22. Barnard, Julian, *Bach Flower Remedies: Form & Function,* Flower Remedy Programme, Hereford, England, 2002.

23. See Miller, Douglas, ed., trans, *Goethe: The Collected Works, Volume 12: Scientific Studies,* Princeton University Press, Princeton, NJ, 1995.

24. See Steiner, Rudolf, *Nature's Open Secret,* SteinerBooks, Great Barrington, MA, 2000.

25. Available online at www.flowersociety.org/twelve.htm.

26. Bach, Edward, *Free Thyself,* published in Barnard, Julian, *Collected Writings of Edward Bach,* Ashgrove Press, London, 1999, page 104.

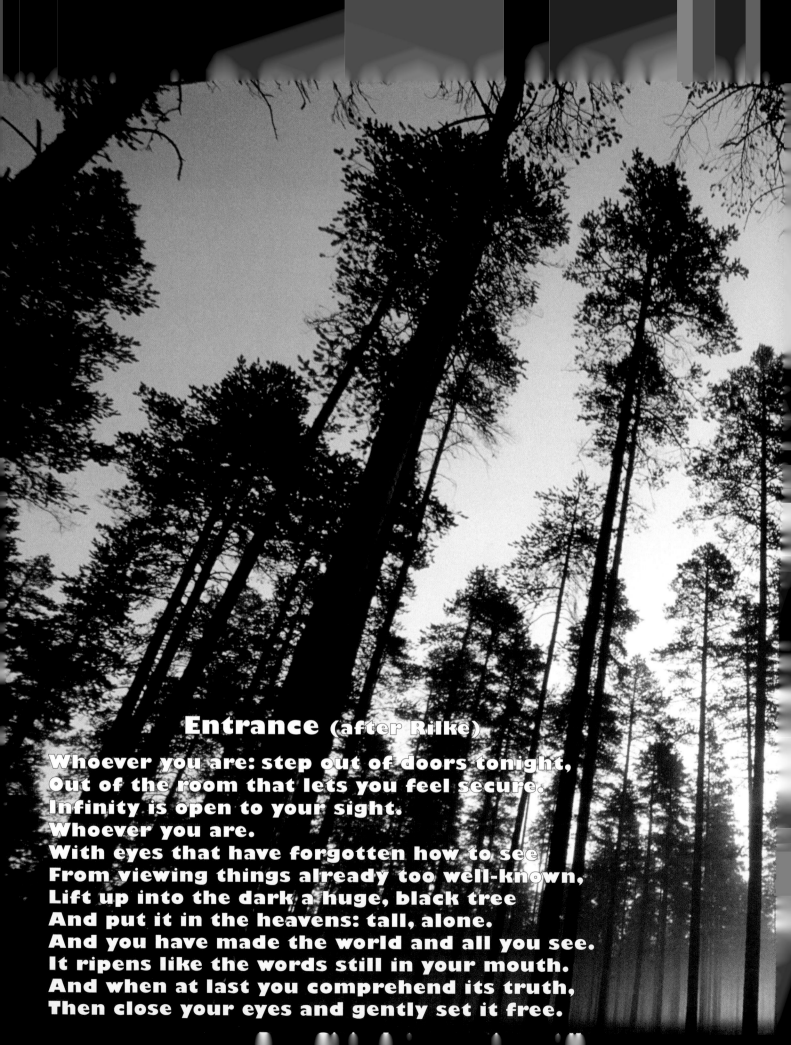

Entrance (after Rilke)

Whoever you are: step out of doors tonight,
Out of the room that lets you feel secure.
Infinity is open to your sight.
Whoever you are.
With eyes that have forgotten how to see
From viewing things already too well-known,
Lift up into the dark a huge, black tree
And put it in the heavens: tall, alone.
And you have made the world and all you see.
It ripens like the words still in your mouth.
And when at last you comprehend its truth,
Then close your eyes and gently set it free.

The Living Science of Nature:

A Foundation for Flower Essence Therapy

by Richard Katz and Patricia Kaminski

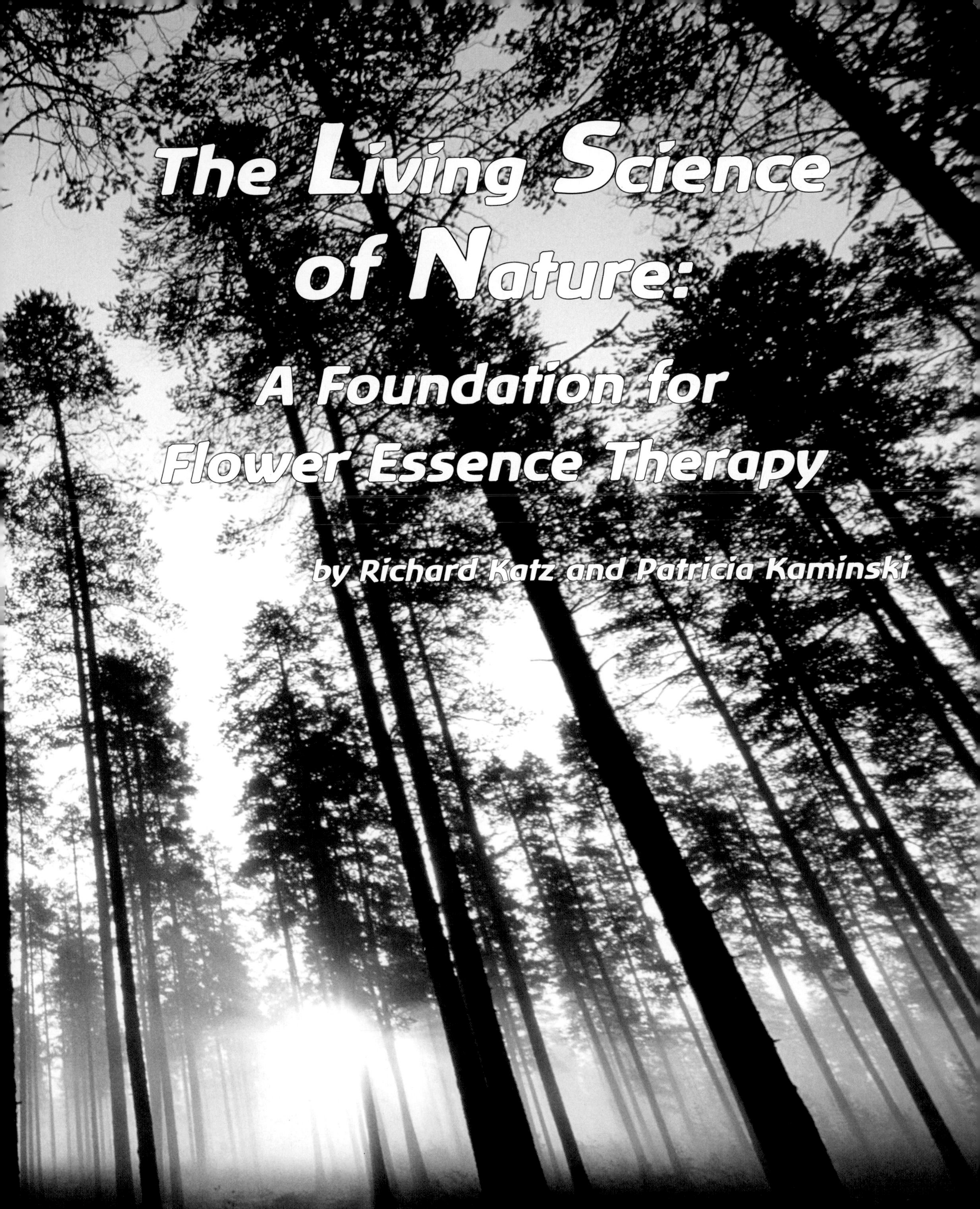

Scots Pine
Pinus sylvestris

The Challenge of Flower Essence Therapy for Science

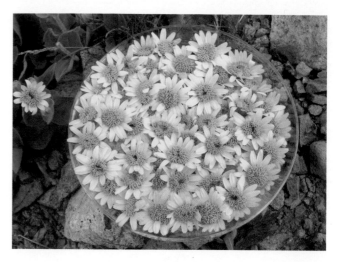

Mother essence of *Arnica mollis*.

How is it possible that a few drops from dilute infusions of wildflowers can catalyze profound benefits for body and soul wellness?

According to the biochemical medical paradigm, nothing should happen. A dosage bottle prepared from the second dilution of the mother essence contains approximately 1/62,000th of the original mother essence, insufficient for standard chemical analysis.

By conventional measurement, flower essences are no more than water and brandy preservative. Since the vibrational imprint of each flower essence cannot be measured by current laboratory instruments, it is assumed that flower essences are bogus. Any healing effects can only be explained as a "placebo." The comment of Dr. Victor Herbert of the National Council Against Health Fraud is typical: "It's a pure fraud. It's been a fraud for 40 years. The only effect the product can have is the effect of the alcohol in it, because there's nothing else in it but water."[1]

However, this explanation contradicts decades of clinical observation and evidence. Thousands of professional practitioners and home-caretakers around the world report significant changes with flower essences. These remedies are also markedly effective with infants, animals, and even plants—cases wherein self-suggestion or mental bias are not operative. Double-blind studies and clinical research[2] demonstrate that flower essences have real effects, although a typical biochemical mechanism cannot be defined. Traditional scientists would probably conclude that any evidence must be false, as did the British journal *Nature,* when Benveniste showed the effects of ultra-dilute homeopathic remedies on microorganisms.[3]

A new paradigm is needed to encompass the evidence. In fact, the prevailing materialistic viewpoint no longer reflects what scientists themselves have discovered in the fields of relativity and quantum physics. The old Newtonian physics presents a strictly mechanistic paradigm, describing concrete objects influenced by external forces in precise, quantifiable, and predicable patterns. But a more advanced physics shows that our world is far more complex, governed by wave-particle duality, the uncertainty principle, energy fields, time-space relativity, and chaos theory. Physicists such as Capra and Bohm have postulated a "new physics" that parallels various *meta*physical teachings of ancient wisdom.[4] Some researchers have begun to explore a theory for the efficacy of "vibrational medicine"[5] by applying quantum physics principles to an understanding of the larger energy fields and life systems that influence physical matter.

Yet, for the most part, the life sciences—and especially medical science—have developed quite narrowly along the path of reductionism, in which feelings, thoughts and experiences are equated with biochemical and electrical mechanisms. Life itself is defined in terms of genetic programming, determined by a cybernetic code of DNA molecules. By limiting its study to what is measurable and quantifiable through mechanical instrumentation, reductionist science ignores *quality* for *quantity;* it measures behavior and ignores experience. If the quantifiable realm ruled by mechanical laws is the only dimension recognized, then machine-like aspects of the human being are the only ones that will be seen. Wear gray glasses, and the world looks gray. If human beings are seen as machines, albeit very complex ones, then healing becomes a mechanical imperative to repair or replace parts, or reprogram the "control system" of DNA molecules and brain chemistry. This is the fallacy of scientific reductionism. It reduces the definition of reality to fit the method of research.

Flower essence therapy—along with other life energy modalities such as homeopathy and acupuncture—challenge the reductionist scientific paradigm. These healing approaches operate through an energetic dimension not fully explained by biochemical mechanisms. Flower essence preparations tap into a much larger force field surrounding each plant, transmitting these qualities to the human energy field. To understand its efficacy, we are challenged to develop a paradigm of living science that encompasses the multidimensionality of the human being and Nature.

Applying Scientific Standards to Flower Essence Therapy

Measuring Unconventional Phenomena

There are various scientific approaches that can be used to evaluate flower essence therapy. The most basic, involves a *conventional* scientific standard that is tapped to measure *unconventional* phenomena. For example, Dr. Jeffrey Cram used the standard double-blind placebo method to measure quantifiable effects of flower essences for stress and environmental sensitivity.[6] The results were documented by measuring sEMG (surface electromyography to measure electrical impulses associated with muscular activity) and EEG (electroencephalogram to show electrical brain wave activity).

The selected instruments were able to measure and quantify electrical activity as a by-product of much deeper soul activity that cannot be captured by such mechanical instruments. Nevertheless, these measurements are a rudimentary way of verifying that flower essences *are* affecting the subjects. Prior scientific research confirms that muscle and brain electrical activity is correlated with certain physiological and psychological experiences, so we can draw further inferences from the results. Such information is a valuable demonstration of how highly dilute flower essences can have effects that are detectable and quantifiable, even though the source of the healing and the actual phenomena are not revealed. It is as if we are following the footprints of an invisible man as he walks through the snow. We have evidence he exists and has crossed our path, but we have not developed the ability to communicate with or perceive him directly.

Clinical Research

Another form of scientific study involves clinical research into flower essence therapy. These studies gather quantifiable data that is analyzed statistically through a professional inventory of symptoms and an evaluative questionnaire distributed to qualified practitioners. The ***FES Depression Study***[7] exemplifies such an approach, using the Beck and Hamilton depression inventories, as does the study by Elizabeth Heyns on midlife crisis and menopause,[8] which uses the Zung

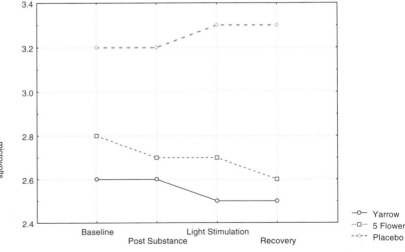

sEMG readings (averaged) from Dr. Cram's study of the effects on flower essences on light sensitivity[6]

Scale for Depression, and the Rojas Scale for Anxiety.

Statistical clinical data is frequently supplemented by qualitative observations and comments from the subjects/patients and researchers/therapists. While a reductionist approach would dismiss non-quantitative data as "anecdotal," it is in fact what makes any analysis possible. Also, general insights regarding therapeutic phenomena that are significant to flower essence practice can be derived from practitioner cases, reports, and interviews. For example, the four stages of flower essence response and the eight "meta-flora" levels of soul healing described by Patricia Kaminski[9] were based upon the analysis of hundreds of case reports and in-depth interviews with numerous practitioners around the world, over the span of approximately two decades.

someone, it may be useful to know that person's height and weight, but these measurements do not give us the full picture of the soul being standing before us. To study the multi-dimensional reality of subtle healing, a fuller methodology is required. This means that the researcher must be in a *relationship* with what is being observed.

Intimacy between the observer and the phenomena to be observed is anathema to scientific orthodoxy. Only a strict "spectator consciousness" is believed to ensure scientific objectivity. However, Heisenberg's Principle of Uncertainty,[10] as outlined in quantum physics, proves that radical separation is illusory. The very act of observation affects that which is observed. Subject and object are intrinsically linked. This scientific discovery from the early part of the twentieth century has yet to penetrate the mainstream of natural science,

> *That my perception be not separated from things … that my perception itself be thinking, my thinking perception.*
> — Johann von Goethe

If the instruments are well-designed and administered, statistical studies provide measurements that are reliable and consistent. On the other hand, it is relatively easy for unskilled or naive practitioners to "contaminate" perceptions through personal projection, or incomplete observation. The answer is not to narrow clinical research to statistical measurements. Rather, we are challenged to hone our observational skills so that practitioners can become precise in studying flower essences and their effects — to develop a qualitative science that is as "objective" as quantitative analysis. Such a conscientious approach to research provides documentation and insight that are valuable in themselves, and certainly as important as quantitative analysis.

Can Natural Science be Holistic?

The *Flower Essence Society* actively promotes studies that can validate flower essence therapy according to accepted scientific standards. Still, quantitative instruments will capture only the quantitative aspects of phenomena. When we meet

which still holds to the paradigm of the detached researcher who has no relationship to the phenomena being observed.

The need for a new method of study that accounts for the heightened consciousness and attunement of the observer with the phenomena observed is especially necessary for plant life. As long as plants are considered as abstract objects to be measured and analyzed in bio-mechanical systems, the properties that make flower essences possible cannot be recognized. As long as we human beings are defined only as bio-mechanical systems, the faculties of subtle perception that foster a relationship with living forces in plants will not be developed. Many people feel this alienation from Nature in the modern world, and seek greater wholeness and unity. It is important that we gain a brief overview of the historical development of the human relationship with Nature, and in particular, the development of plant science and taxonomy. In this way, we can appreciate the need to develop a living science of flower essence therapy.

A Historical Perspective on Plant Science

Ancient Humanity

For most of humanity's past there was no science, as there was no sense of individuality separate from the social or natural environment. Science could only arise when human beings felt themselves as distinct from Nature, and thus could stand back as observers, study it, and develop a conscious relationship with it. Human beings possessed a direct clairvoyance based upon the ability to feel the qualities of other living beings as an inner experience. For example, the healing properties of plants were known not by a modern method of analysis, nor simply by naive trial and error (as conventional wisdom suggests), but by entering into the life of the plant, experiencing its inner nature and the celestial forces that formed it. Ancient humanity experienced a world that was permeated by creative forces and beings. The stars and planets were not just distant points of light in the night sky, but sources of palpable spiritual influence shaping life on Earth.[11]

When seers such as Edgar Cayce[12] and Rudolf Steiner[13] examined the conditions of our ancient world (often thought of as the prehistoric civilizations of Lemuria and Atlantis), they discovered a vastly different reality than the one we inhabit today. The earth was softer, more fluid, and more permeable to archetypal formative forces. The physical forms of the earth—mineral, plant, animal, and human—were likewise more flexible and responsive to environmental influences. As the earth evolved, it became harder, and more fixed. Human consciousness also began to contract and harden, by forming a *sense of Self* separate from the spiritual and natural world. Gradually, only highly trained or unusual persons, who still possessed a residue of the old clairvoyant faculties, were able to perceive the bridge between earthly and cosmic reality. Thus, there developed the extraordinary role of the shaman, or medicine woman or man, who kept alive a supersensible knowledge of the plant world.

As human consciousness further individuated, the power of individuating thought began to awaken. Human beings started to regard themselves as separate from Nature. Consequently, direct perception and relationship with the supersensible aspect of Nature was diminished. Instinctive knowledge of plants faded into memory, and was preserved in folklore. Yet, the development of humanity's individuated consciousness was also a step forward in human evolution. Awakening from a dream-like unity with Nature, human beings began to clarify sense perceptions, and reflect on the meaning of what was perceived, developing new creative powers of soul. These new thinking faculties were gradually applied to the study of Nature, through the dawning powers of observation and reasoning.

The Beginnings of Botany: The Neolithic Revolution

One of the first sciences to emerge from the primordial dream was the study of plants, what is termed *botany* today.[14] Unfortunately, for many people the science of botany has the feeling of a dry and stuffy academic pursuit, burdened by arcane disputes about the proper names of plants. Yet, botany, and particularly botanical *taxonomy* (from the Greek *taxis*, meaning "arrangement"), can provide us with a wealth of knowledge about the nature of plants. Married to holistic science, botany provides many important keys for appreciating flower essence qualities.

It is important to acquire a brief overview of the evolution of plant science alongside changes in human consciousness. The first conscious study of plants occurred with the development of agriculture, sometimes called the "Neolithic revolution," about 10,000 years ago. Ancient Mesopotamian and Persian cultures reached extraordinary levels of development, including elaborate gardens wherein human ingenuity worked co-creatively with the elemental kingdoms. Plant knowledge also developed as medicinal knowledge, especially in ancient Egypt, Babylonia, and China. The first botanical studies were grounded in an intimate working relationship with plants, particularly among women

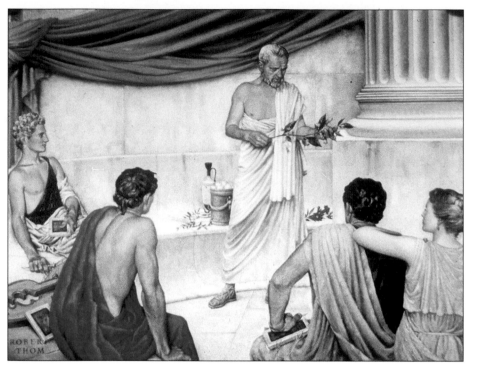

Anaximander, a pupil of Thales, was first to systematically study living organisms in about 520 BC. Approximately two centuries later, Aristotle's pupil **Theophrastus** was first to fully develop botanical studies. A major question considered by Aristotle and Theophrastus involved the characteristics most suitable to differentiate one plant from another (*differentiae*), and which naturally relate plants to one another (*affines*). They wanted to know if a classification system was merely an *artificial way* of cataloguing for convenient reference, or whether it was based on *natural relationships* in which an inherent *Idea* or *Archetype* could be revealed by comparing and contrasting its various physical manifestations. This question is still a valid one for botanists more than twenty-five hundred years later.

in their roles as gardeners, cooks, herbalists, and healers. It was a practical science, concerned with recognizing and distinguishing plants useful for food and medicine. These contributions were a transition—the old faculties of direct sensing of Nature were beginning to fade, and the intellectual faculties which would allow an exact objective science had yet to be developed.

Greek Nature Philosophy

"Modern" botanical science was born in Greece, during approximately the sixth century B.C., when philosophical thinking first developed, and human cognition began to organize perceptions of Nature. Greek *philosophy* was not the dry, speculative pursuit we might think of today, rather it was literally the *love for Sophia*, the spiritual being from whom Nature Wisdom emanated. Philosophic inquiry was a method of soul initiation through the Greek mystery schools. Striving to understand and commune with the Creator Beings who shaped the living earth, Greek philosophy was a profound and intense pursuit to discover the nature of reality. Especially important was the ability to perceive the world of cosmic Ideas, or archetypes, from which the beauty and majesty of the natural world derived its sacred power and meaning.

Following what he believed was a "natural" classification, Theophrastus sub-divided plants as trees, shrubs, under-shrubs, and herbs. Many distinctions were noted such as monocotyledons and dicotyledons, radial and bilateral symmetry, annuals and perennials. Natural groupings of plants were outlined, such as lilies, umbels, legumes, grasses, conifers, catkin-bearing trees, thistles, and palms. The studies of Theophrastus were the precursor for Linnaeus' system many centuries later. He also studied plant morphology (structure and shape) and ecology (its relation to the environment). Greek scientific tradition did not contain the element of experimentation as in modern science, but did develop systematic observation of natural phenomena, and the use of the rational mind to appreciate the creative forces and laws of growth that characterized the natural world.

Greek botanical tradition was maintained for a while by the Romans such as Pliny and Galen, but no longer nourished by the mystery wisdom of the Greek philosophical schools. After the fall of Rome and the ensuing "Dark Ages," the active pursuit of botanical knowledge atrophied in Europe. Remnants of Greek botanical knowledge were preserved in the Arabic centers of learning and medicine, leading to the practical development of pharmacology. In the medieval monasteries of Europe, old Greek botanical texts were copied by rote, including the reproduction of plant drawings many centuries old. But without a real relationship to the natural world, the resemblance to actual living plants became less and less apparent.

Medieval woodcut of an Ash tree

Meanwhile, a parallel evolution of botany occurred in China, around the 6th century BC. Highly sophisticated botanical texts and medicinal herbals were produced, based on meticulous plant observation. Although the Chinese herbal and botanical tradition lacked the philosophical depth of the Greek mystery schools, or the precision of modern botany, it had the advantage of profound living wisdom and experience based upon two millennia of unbroken tradition.

The European Renaissance and the Linnaean System of Taxonomy

When the renewal of direct inquiry into the natural world surfaced during the European Renaissance, the works of Theophrastus were re-discovered, and stimulated an inquiry into plants which were actually observed in Nature. Pressed and dried specimens were prepared for study, and real-istic illustrations of plants drawn from live specimens replaced the copies of medieval manuscripts. This development of more exact perceptions and representations of plant specimens paralleled the increasing individuation of human consciousness. As human beings continued to develop as distinct entities in relation to the social and natural world around them, they could then stand back and observe that world with greater clarity and precision.

One of the first major early Renaissance botanists was **Andrea Cesalpino** (1519-1603) of Italy, who based his classification system on the fruit of the plant as its most fundamental nature. Other botanists added the flower, and considered the whole reproductive process of the plant as its most distinguishing feature. Observation and description of the external mechanisms of plant fertilization was spurred by Leeuwenhoek's development of the microscope in the 17th century. An obsessive interest in the mechanics of plant reproduction led scientists to liken their investigations to those of animal sexuality. For example, they assumed that the pollen from the flower stamens reached the pistils and fertilized the ovary through a similar male-female polarity that is observed in the animal world.

Carolus **Linnaeus**[15] (Swedish name, Carl von Linné, 1707-1778) is well known as the originator of the currently accepted system of botanical classification. In fact, he built his system on the work of many previous botanists, going back all the way to Theophrastus. Linnaeus' greatest contribution was that of an organizer. By the force of his intention, and his great skill in plant observation, he succeeded in establishing a single, universally accepted taxonomy.

Linnaeus

The basis of Linnaeus' system is the concept of the genus, a grouping of plants sharing a common reproductive (flower and fruit) structure. Within each genus are found a number of species, which are often distinguished by non-reproductive characters such as leaf structure, but which must be genetically distinct, in that they reproduce true to type. Previous to Linnaeus, the genus name was often used to describe the main, or first discovered plant in that classification, with *specific* descriptive phrases added to the name to distinguish various other species in the genus. This became unwieldy, not only because of the length of the resulting names, but also because these descriptive phrases needed continual revision as new species were discovered. For example, one wild morning glory wound up with the name *Convolvulus argenteus foliis ovatis divisis basi truncatis: laciniis intermediis duplo longioribus.*

Linnaeus' solution, now the basis of modern botanical classification, was to assign a single name to distinguish a species. This name may be a descriptive word, but could just as likely be the Latinized name of a person who discovered it. The species name, preceded by the name of the genus in

which the plant is found, comprises its official botanical name. Thus, Linnaeus' system is called the *binomial* (two name) system of classification, offering an international language of plant identification that spans barriers of nationality and culture. For example, the wild morning glory, known as "Bindweed," is designated as *Convolvulus arvensis.*

The genus and species form only a part of a complex classification system of hierarchical relationships in Nature. Starting from the broadest categories (but leaving out several intermediate levels), we have the Kingdoms of Nature (such as Plant and Animal); then within the Plant Kingdom are various Subkingdoms, Superdivisions and Divisions, including algae and fungi; mosses and liverworts; ferns and related plants; gymnosperms and true flowering plants (Magnoliophyta or Anthopytya, also known as the

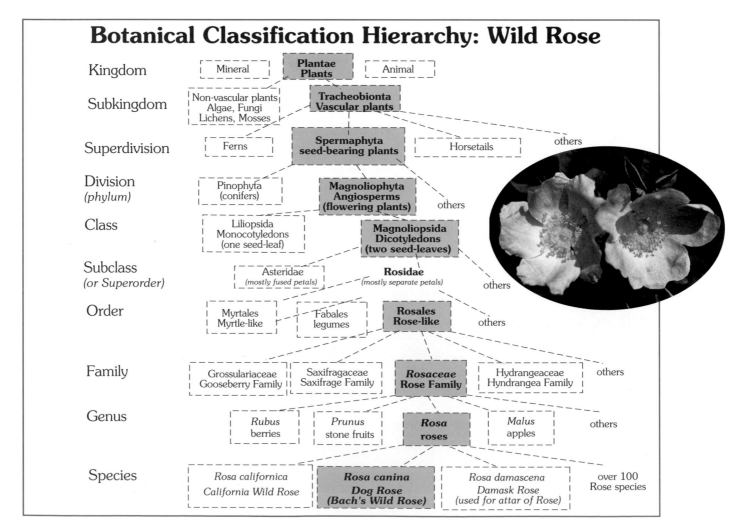

Botanical Classification Hierarchy: Wild Rose

Kingdom	Mineral	**Plantae Plants**	Animal	
Subkingdom	Non-vascular plants Algae, Fungi Lichens, Mosses	**Tracheobionta Vascular plants**		
Superdivision	Ferns	**Spermaphyta seed-bearing plants**	Horsetails	others
Division *(phylum)*	Pinophyta (conifers)	**Magnoliophyta Angiosperms (flowering plants)**	others	
Class	Liliopsida Monocotyledons (one seed-leaf)	**Magnoliopsida Dicotyledons (two seed-leaves)**		
Subclass *(or Superorder)*	Asteridae *(mostly fused petals)*	**Rosidae** *(mostly separate petals)*	others	
Order	Myrtales Myrtle-like / Fabales legumes	**Rosales Rose-like**	others	
Family	Grossulariaceae Gooseberry Family / Saxifragaceae Saxifrage Family	***Rosaceae Rose Family***	Hydrangeaceae Hyndrangea Family	others
Genus	*Rubus* berries / *Prunus* stone fruits	***Rosa roses***	*Malus* apples	others
Species	*Rosa californica* California Wild Rose	***Rosa canina Dog Rose (Bach's Wild Rose)***	*Rosa damascena* Damask Rose *(used for attar of Rose)*	over 100 Rose species

Angiosperms). Within the Division of flowering plants are two Classes of Monocotyledons (Magnoliopsida) and Dicotyledons (Magnoliopsida), having one and two seed leaves respectively. We then have Subclasses and Orders; for example, within the dicotyledons we have rose-like plants (Rosales). Each Order is a grouping of plant Families; for example the Rose Family or Rosaceae. Some large families, such as the Asteraceae (Sunflower Family) are further divided into Tribes. There are variations in the contemporary Linnaean classification system among different botanical authorities. *(References in this article are based upon the work of Cronquist[16], one of the more commonly used systems.)*

Finally, we come to the plant genus and species, which constitute the scientific binomials of plants. For example, the Rose Family contains such genera as *Rubus* (many of the berries), *Prunus* (fruit and nut trees such as cherry, plum, and almond), and *Rosa* (wild and horticultural roses). The species name then distinguishes plants within the same genus. For example, Almond is *Prunus amygdalus*, while Apricot is *Prunus armeniaca*, and the Bach Cherry Plum is *Prunus cerasifera*. Further distinctions are sometimes made through subspecies and varieties, such as Nectarine (*Prunus persica* var. *nectarina).* To write a full botanical name, the botanist who first authored the name is appended to the binomial. Thus the Dog Rose developed as a flower essence by Dr. Bach is *Rosa canina* Linnaeus.

The Linnaean system forms the basis of modern botanical nomenclature. Although it has been modified and expanded over the last two-and-a-half centuries, its essential outline remains intact. It is a highly structured universal language for differentiating, naming, and arranging plant species. Linnaeus' book *Species Plantarium,* published in 1753, is still considered the starting date for the classification system used today. While Linnaeus' system is successful as an international method of nomenclature, its drawback is that it obscures the living relationship between plant phenomena and the overarching cosmic archetypes that Greek philosophers had so ardently championed.

Modern Influences: Phenotype and Genotype

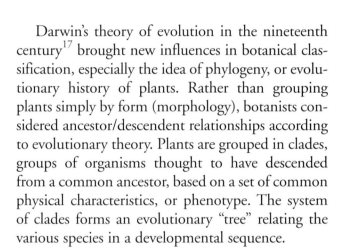

The trend in modern botanical science is to give increasing emphasis to abstract nomenclature derived from the computer analyses of DNA molecules, rather than an actual encounter with living plants.

Darwin's theory of evolution in the nineteenth century[17] brought new influences in botanical classification, especially the idea of phylogeny, or evolutionary history of plants. Rather than grouping plants simply by form (morphology), botanists considered ancestor/descendent relationships according to evolutionary theory. Plants are grouped in clades, groups of organisms thought to have descended from a common ancestor, based on a set of common physical characteristics, or phenotype. The system of clades forms an evolutionary "tree" relating the various species in a developmental sequence.

Today, many botanists are turning to molecular biology, and computer analysis for classification. Taxonomists now consider the genotype, a set of genetic characteristics considered to determine the organism's physical characteristics (phenotype). This development has accelerated in the last half-century, with the mapping of the structure of the DNA molecule and its sequences of nucleotides, considered by reductionist science as the structural "secret of life."[18] Proposals for reordering the Linnaean-based systems[19], have been promoted by the Angiosperm Phylogeny Group[20], and most recently by the Green Plant Phylogeny Research Coordination Group, or "Deep Green",[21] located at the University of California, Berkeley, and funded by a grant from the U.S. National Science Foundation, Department of Agriculture and Energy Department. A related group at U.C. Berkeley, called "Deep Gene," is promoting the "integration of plant phylogenetics and plant genomics."[22]

Reductionism: The Failure to Find Meaning and Context in Nature

The trend in modern botanical science is to give increasing emphasis to abstract nomenclature derived from the computer analyses of DNA molecules, rather than experiencing an actual encounter with living plants. No one has seen the supposed phylogenetic trees of evolution. They are, in fact, hypothetical constructions that attempt to explain the basis of creation through DNA phenomena. The foundation of genuine science has always been careful observation of actual phenomena in the physical world. In many ways, the lack of relationship to the natural world is another version of the "Dark Ages," when botanists became blind from the real world of Nature around them.

Craig Holdrege, founder and director of the Nature Institute[23], challenges the reductionist dogma of contemporary genetic science:[24]

> What a gene "is" is dependent on the organism in its spatially and temporally unfolding existence. You always have to presuppose the organism to understand the gene. This conclusion has far-reaching implications.
>
> Take, for example, our conception of evolutionary processes. The scenario taught in schools and universities around the world is: the gradual accumulation of gene mutations causes organisms to evolve new characteristics. But this scenario doesn't work, if we take the results of developmental genetics seriously. Rather, we must imagine the evolving organism utilizing "old" genes in new ways to realize new evolutionary developmental characteristics. This view removes genes from their pedestal in evolutionary theory, since they can no longer be seen as the driving evolutionary force. The whole organism — which has been virtually lost in genetic and evolutionary thinking today — returns to the center stage of development and evolution.[25]

Henri Bortoff argues in *The Wholeness of Nature,*[26] that all scientific investigation filters phenomena through an organizing principle or value system. If we live in an economic system based on competition, we see the natural world based on "survival of the fittest." If we live in a world of man-made machines, we see living organisms as mechanisms with interchangeable parts. If we look at the world through a microscope, we see organisms as simply the sum of their molecules. If we crystallize living tissues for chemical analyses, we see chemical structures that seem to determine life processes. If we use computers to analyze genetic traits and build phylogenetic trees, then we see the genetic material as a kind of computer code which programs the form and behavior of living organisms.

The question then becomes, what is the filter through which we view Nature? What is it that we value in Nature, or why should Nature have meaning for us? From this perspective, we can see that scientific reductionism is akin to a type of nihilism that shortchanges the natural world of any true meaning and context. Consider this analogy: a group of scientists from another planet discover the ruins of a building containing shelves filled with square objects. The scientists have clever intellectual faculties and construct a detailed inventory of their discovery. They describe thin sheets of cellulose bound together with thicker cellulose covers. The cellulose sheets are covered with a series of shapes. These shapes are analyzed by a statistical program for frequency and patterns of repetition. No meaning can be found. However, a chemical analysis of the cellulose reveals a low burning point. Therefore the archeologists conclude that this is a fuel depot, for a primitive form of energy production.

Suppose we knew what the archeologists had actually found was a library of books. Unfortunately, they cannot appreciate the language contained in these books, nor do they have any concept of what a book is. This ignorance leads them to reduce what they discover to physical measurements and utilitarian meaning. A book cannot be understood unless its meaning can be read. It is more than its sheer physical constituents, *it is the embodiment of creative ideas in a physical form.* Similarly, if we can no longer see the physical realm of Nature as an expression of living Creation, embodying meaning, purpose and qualities, then our perception of Nature becomes more and more myopic, ultimately reduced to physical molecules or genetic structures.

A Holistic Science of Nature

The Alchemical Tradition

Alchemy is often dismissed as primitive fantasy, attempting for example, to create gold out of lead. The real alchemical tradition is actually a far more complex path of knowledge. It is based upon a dynamic and revolutionary understanding of the human being and Nature. The natural world is viewed not as a mere collection of objects for study, but as a *living script*, full of meaning and significance, reaching its fullest potential when consciously appreciated by the human individuality.

Alchemy had its origins in the ancient Egyptian civilization, when the great initiate **Toth** (known to the Greeks as **Hermes Trismegistos**) taught that Nature is an embodiment of divine principles, summarized "As Above, So Below." The earth was not viewed as separate from the spiritual world, but uniquely integral to the whole of creative expression. Alchemical teachings were developed in unique ways in many parts of the world including China, Japan, and ancient Persia.

Alchemy was given new development and emphasis through the Rosicrucian spiritual order, founded by **Christian Rosenkreutz**[27] (1378-1484). At a time when medieval theology prescribed an other-worldly religion, the Rosicrucians followed a path of discovering the spirit through a knowledge of Nature. Based on the ancient Hermetic teachings, the Rosicrucians knew that the microcosm of the human being reflected the macrocosmic reality of Nature. Such understanding formed the basis for the tradition of alchemy.

The herbalist/physician **Paracelsus**[28] (1493-1541) was strongly influenced by Rosicrucian/alchemical thinking. He formulated his well-known "Doctrine of Signatures," showing how the perceptible forms of plants were clues to healing qualities. Resemblances between plant parts and human anatomy often indicated therapeutic use, as in the hairy leaves of Comfrey or Mullein used for the intestines or lungs, with their hair-like villi, or the capillary-like structures of Red Clover

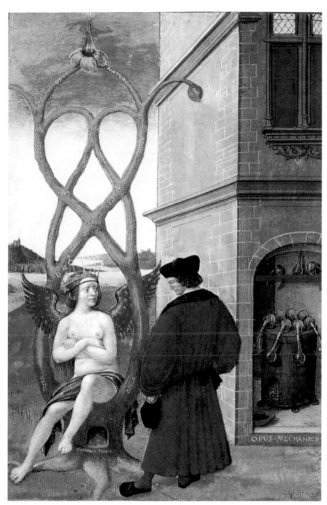

Alchemical illustration by Jehan Perreal, Austria, 1516. Mercury is the winged guardian of the alchemical caduceus, with a flower at the apex. He advises the alchemist to leave his mechanical laboratory and follow a spiralic route of transformation, akin to that of the plant.

There is a rich alternative scientific tradition which supports a soul-spiritual perception of Nature. It is not based upon a return to the dream clairvoyance of humanity's ancient past. Rather, it is an approach that utilizes the clear perception and logical thought that science offers, but extends the realms of perceiving and thinking beyond present-day boundaries. The foundation for such a path begins with alchemical thought and culminates in the holistic natural science of Johann von Goethe.

blossoms for blood purification. The habitat and growth patterns of plants was also intensively considered as a means of understanding their healing properties.

Famous herbalists like **John Gerard**[29] (1545-1612) and **Nicholas Culpeper**[30] (1616-1654), extended the Doctrine of Signatures beyond the physical form to include celestial influences. Even such noted early physical scientists as **Johannes Kepler**[31] (1571-1630), famous for his calculations of planetary orbits, had a deep reverence for spiritual beings and forces that influenced astronomical phenomena. Unfortunately, Rosicrucian/alchemical thinking was soon eclipsed, as scientific thinking hardened into a more narrowly materialistic mode, with the goal of manipulating Nature for utilitarian human purposes.

Goethe: The Art of Natural Science

Johann Wolfgang von Goethe[32] (1749-1832), better known for his literary masterpiece *Faust*, gave the impetus for a living approach to scientific study, only now beginning to receive greater recognition. During a sojourn in Italy, Goethe observed a great variety of plant life previously unfamiliar to him. He developed a revolutionary theory of plant metamorphosis, along with a compelling theory of color dynamics that challenges the prevailing Newtonian perspective. Goethe also made significant discoveries in geology, and animal and human anatomy. Goethe's botanical work points the way to holistic science, as disciplined and systematic as conventional scientific research, while also a path of inner development and metaphysical perception.

At the basis of Goethe's scientific activity is the cognition of living "Ideas" within the phenomena of Nature. Disparate perceptions are organized into larger relationships and meaning. Goethe understood that we first need to cognize what all plants have in common. He points to an embracing archetypal plant, called the *Urpflanze,* as the creative source of all possible plants, even ones which have not yet appeared in Nature. The image-making activity that helps grasp the concept of the *Urpflanze* as "primal phenomena" leads the experience of the "time body" of the plant as its most essential gesture. All plants live in a weaving, dynamic field of life energy. They are united by their capacity for continuous *metamorphosis* through expansion and contraction: the breaking open of the seed into leaf, the enhancement of green leafy growth, the in-breath that creates the calyx, the cosmic fulfillment of the flower, the contraction into pollen, the final expansion into seed-bearing fruit, and the seed that completes the life cycle.

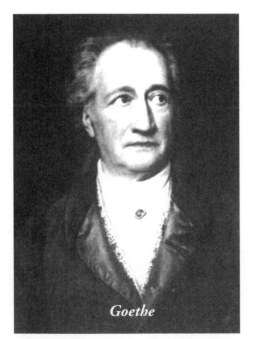

Goethe

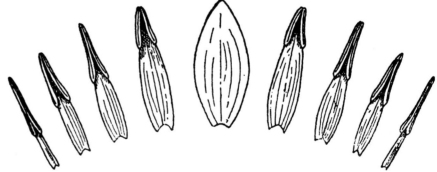

Goethe's drawing of the successive transformation of petals into stamens in the white water lily, Nymphaea alba. *This simple sketch shows a principle of plant metamorphosis that Goethe found repeatedly in all stages of plant growth: a central unifying principle through which expansion and contraction occur over time. Perception of the plant's movement in time allows us to grasp the etheric dimension of fluid life process.*

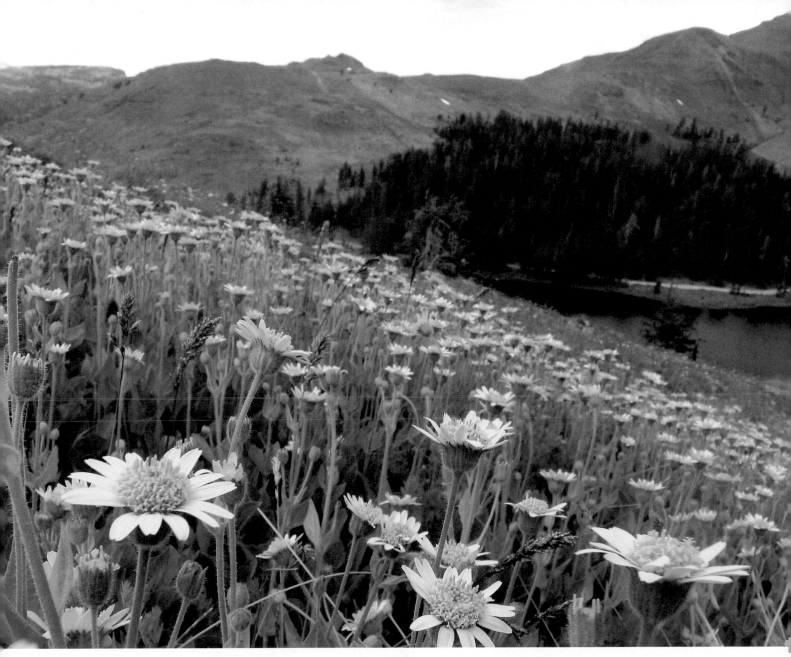

Field of **Arnica mollis** *in the high Sierra Nevada mountains.*

Nature! We are surrounded and embraced by her: powerless to separate ourselves from her, and powerless to penetrate beyond her.

Without asking, or warning, she snatches us up into her circling dance, and whirls us on until we are tired, and drop from her arms.

She is ever shaping new forms: what is, has never yet been;
what has been, comes not again.
Everything is new, and yet naught but the old.

from *Nature*, by Johann Goethe

The ability to engage the perception to behold metamorphic stages of plant growth is more than an intellectual "fact." Its truth is an active form of "science meditation." It can only be appreciated through inner participation — the ability to breathe with and inwardly imagine each stage of the plant's expression as a dynamic, living reality. As the *Urpflanze* illumines the soul's perception, it becomes both an inward perception and a bridge to the outer beholding of all plants in Nature.

Once the fluid "etheric" experience of the *Urpflanze* is mastered, then each individual variation can be appreciated with great clarity and sensitivity. We learn to look upon plants not merely as physical, static matter, but as dynamic, ever-changing forms. Within these forms however, we can see that each plant has a unique expression, or gesture. As we live into a plant like the sunflower, we can see that it begins its rapid growth in the heat of the summer, turning its face sunward, producing a bright yellow seed head on its towering stalk, before bending down to earth. By contrast, the sweet violet blooms in the cool damp of early spring, its small purple flower remaining close to the earth, exuding a delicate sweet fragrance. Living into each plant as it actually grows in Nature, leads us to develop imagination and perception that is true to the plant itself, not simply our own psychic projection. At the same time, it is a far more living encounter than a chemical analysis or taxonomical classification. When we live with a plant in this manner, with full faculties of the soul brought to the perception, we begin to see that each plant's unique gesture is also a qualitative experience. For example, the sunflower's exultation in the sun shows us a quality of magnanimity and extroversion; the violet's cool color and diminutive presence suggests a quality of containment and purity.

Goethe's methodology resurrects and expands the mystery wisdom of ancient Greek philosophy, which had given the original impetus to botanical science through its striving for inner knowledge of the world. Goethe outlines a way to experience and cognize the etheric laws out of which the created world of Nature arises: the basis for a new kind of clairvoyance that is intelligent and consciously present to the physical world, yet cognizant of other dimensions that give the plant life and form. Although he gave much credit to Linnaeus, Goethe often found the Linnaean system artificial, ignoring profound interrelationships of form and forces which could be directly perceived through an awakened observation of plant life.

Unfortunately, Goethe's remarkable research was largely ignored in the rush of nineteenth century scientific progress. Far more influential was the evolutionary theory of the English scientist **Charles Darwin**[33] (1809-1882), which described the vast variety of living forms in Nature as the outcome of random variations filtered through the sole criteria of survival adaptation.

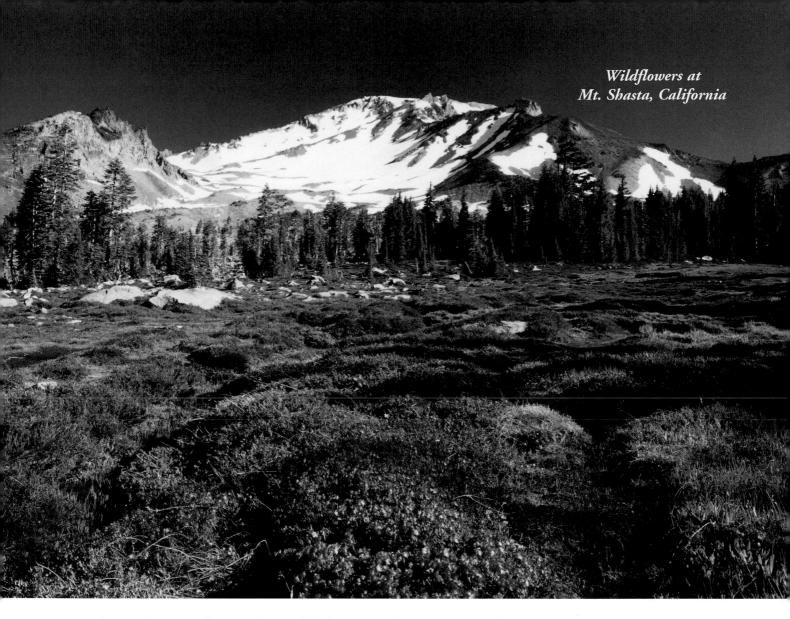

Wildflowers at
Mt. Shasta, California

People walk over the earth and it is a conglomeration of rocks and stones to them, but men must learn to grasp that all surrounding them is the true physical expression for the Spirit of the Earth. Just as the body is ensouled, so is the earth planet the external expression for an indwelling spirit. When men look on the earth as possessing body and soul as man does, only then do they have an idea of what Goethe meant when he said "All things corruptible are but a semblance." When you see tears run down the human countenance you do not examine by the laws of physics how quickly or how slowly the tears roll down; they express to you the inner sadness of the soul, just as the smiling cheek is the expression for the soul's inner joy. The pupil must educate himself to see in each single flower in the meadow he crosses, the outer expression of a living being, the expression of the Spirit dwelling in the Earth. Some flowers seem to be tears, others are the joyful expression of the earth's Spirit. Every stone, every plant, every flower, all is for him the outer expression of the indwelling Earth Spirit, its physiognomy that speaks to him.

Theosophy of the Rosicrucian, by Rudolf Steiner, Chapter XIV

> **Do not look beyond the phenomena; they are the doctrine.** — Johann von Goethe

Rudolf Steiner[34] (1861-1925) rescued Goethe's scientific works from relative obscurity. As a young man, Steiner was given the editorship of the complete edition of Goethe's scientific writings. Later, he developed a comprehensive science of the spirit (Anthroposophy), in which the relationship between sense perception and spiritual cognition is crucial. Scientific study begins with clear sense perception, which is then gradually extended and refined until it is capable of grasping "super-sensible" realms. Such an approach requires recognition of the importance of the living ideas which organize and give meaning to the vast array of percepts with which the scientist works. A living science of Nature forms the basis for Anthroposophic Medicine and Biodynamic Agriculture, initiated by Steiner in 1924. Fundamental to these sciences is an awareness of the Earth as a living organism permeated by spiritual forces which work through the minerals, plants, animals, and elemental kingdoms.

Through the impulses of Goethean science and Anthroposophy, significant new directions have been charted by some modern scientists and mathematicians. For example, *The Plant Between the Sun and Earth,* by **Olive Whicher** and **George Adams**[35], presents projective geometry as a mathematics of the living forces which shape plant growth and metamorphosis. The Scottish mathematician **Lawrence Edwards**[36] made detailed studies of the morphology of plant buds. His research revealed that the geometric shapes of plant buds pulsate regularly in a way that directly correlates to the conjunctions and oppositions of the moon with the plant's traditional ruling planet, thus providing mathematical evidence for the theories of celestial influence popularized by such herbalists as Paracelsus and Culpeper. *The Plant,* by **Gerbert Grohmann**[37], is a brilliant Goethean approach to botanical groupings of plants. In *Healing Plants*, **Wilhelm Pelikan**[38] relates the physical, chemical, morphological, and etheric properties of the plants to their healing properties for Anthroposophic Medicine, as seen within the context of their plant family relationships.

The Practice of Participatory Science

Goethe's methodology is often called "participatory." It recognizes that the subject-object duality of modern science is a false dichotomy. Instead what is required for the true scientist is *active participation in the phenomena,* not through fanciful projection but rather through living thinking and perception. Participatory science offers a systematic path of knowledge with the goal of understanding the lawfulness of Nature. It is holistic and ecological in its ethic, employing a methodology that sees each part of an organism or entity in relation to the whole. This applies not only to structure and form in space, but also to processes in time. This path of science is truly integrative, uniting imaginative thinking with acute and disciplined observation. Nature is the teacher, guiding scientists to "see" her creative, archetypal laws within the actual phenomena. The following are some of the key components of a participatory approach to science:

Direct experience of Nature: This first step is the foundation of participatory science. We best understand natural phenomena by starting with precise *observation*, engaging the senses before attempting to explain our experience with abstractions or intellectual labels. When we look at a pine tree our first inclination is to name it: "That's a pine." By doing so, we have already categorized it, and limited our ability to truly *see* it.

When we behold a pine with open attention, we first note its tall, upright central trunk, with the side branches radiating out in all directions. Unlike the oak, with its spreading horizontal branches, the pine branches swirl in spirals around the central axis of the trunk, forming a conical shape, and coming to a point at the crown. Depending on the species, we may observe that the lower trunk lacks branches, further emphasizing the upward gesture of the tree. Gazing up to the towering crowns of the pine trees, we notice dark green needle-like leaves shimmering in the sun and we can discern pine cones hanging from the branches. If we pick up some fallen cones and examine them closely, we can feel their woody rigidity, quite unlike the delicate flower or luscious fruit of the apple tree, for example. Yet, we are soon struck by the spiralic pattern of the cone, culminating at its apex, echoing the same formative movement we noted in the tree as a whole. Taking a closer look at the pine needles, we see a dominant central vein and a very narrow leaf culminating at a sharp point. The needles are in bundles (two, three, or five depending on the species), and as we hold them in our hands we are aware of a pungent, oily aroma that characterizes a pine forest on a sunny day. Coming closer to the trunk of the tree, we notice the bark is rough with a patchwork pattern full of fissures and breaks. If the tree has been damaged, we may see some of the sap oozing out, forming a resinous scab with its oily aroma.

Forming an inner image: Our experience of the outer phenomena is now re-created within the soul. Goethe calls this faculty "exact imagination." It differs from projection of our wishes or a fanciful imagination that says more about ourselves than what is observed. Exact imagination is true to our encounter with Nature. We need to vividly recreate the picture of the tall pine tree, with its towering trunk and linear leaves, as clearly as if we were looking directly at it. This process takes practice, usually checking back and forth between physical observation and creation with the "soul's eye." We are reminded that Goethe's pioneering work *Metamorphosis of Plants*[39] was not so much a theoretical treatise, rather it outlined his own research with plants, using disciplined observation and exact imagination.

Inward participation in the processes of Nature: The third step in the participatory process guides us toward temporal as well as spatial phenomena, such as the relationship between various parts of a plant, or among various plants. It may also involve a series of observations during the life cycle of the plant. To use Goethe's image, we step into the "dance of Nature" by re-creating the dynamic fields of etheric expression and movement that characterize the plant.

We can animate our imagination of the pine cone by following its spirals to the apex, moving then to the similar spiraling upward movement of the branches, culminating at the tip of the crown, and reaching above to the light. We can imagine a polar opposite movement in the unseen root reaching down towards the center of the earth. As we stretch our imagination over the vast life span of the pine, we see it reaching ever upward, dropping lower branches on the forest floor, along with needles and cones. Moving our attention to the pine needles, we can feel the same quality of linearity we experienced in the trunk.

By creating an analogue of the plant's process as an inner activity, we experience the plant from within ourselves, as well as from our external observations. These activities need not be limited to sight. For example, we can sit with our back against the trunk of the tree and feel the uprightness of our own spine. The aroma of the leaves and

> **By creating an analogue of the plant's process as an inner activity, we experience the plant from within ourselves, as well as from our external observations.**

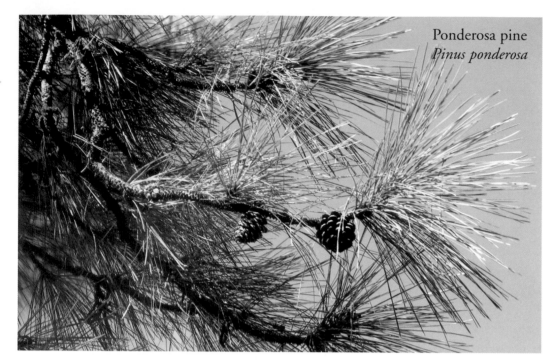

Ponderosa pine
Pinus ponderosa

In the pine, we experience these forces as the upward, light-seeking forces, especially the cleansing warmth embodied in the aromatic oils found in the leaves and sap.

The pine is full of light, especially as we note its silica-rich leaves sparkling in the sun.

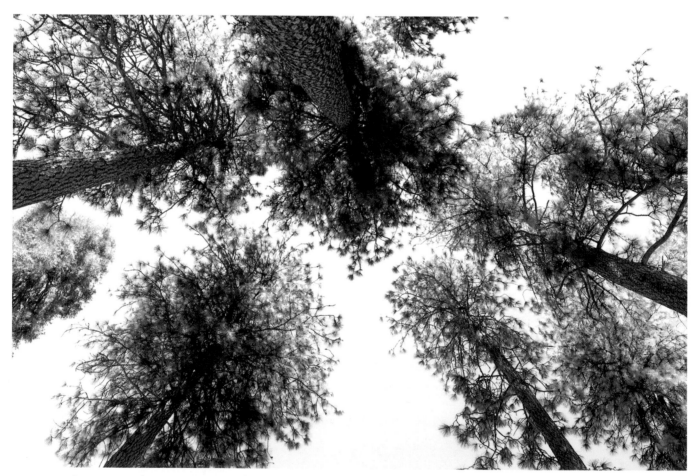

As we visit the pine again and again, we feel its particular radiance. We sense a distinct energetic shift in our own being; a vertical alignment that orients itself to the upward streaming of light.

Ponderosa Pine
Pinus ponderosa

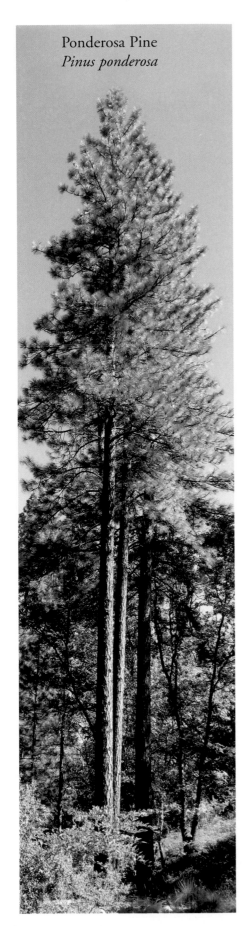

We are struck by the spiralic pattern of the cone, culminating at its apex, echoing the same formative movement we noted in the tree as a whole.

(Spirals shown are "path curves" as depicted in The Vortex of Life, by Lawrence Edwards.[36])

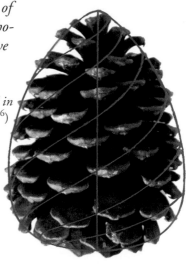

The Pine flower essence brings warmth and uplifting light into the soul, transforming dark, brooding melancholia and excessive attachment to the past.

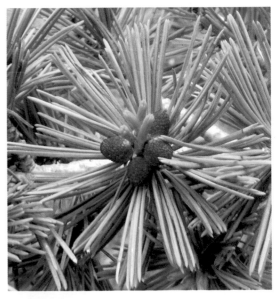

Female flowers of Lodgepole Pine
Pinus contorta

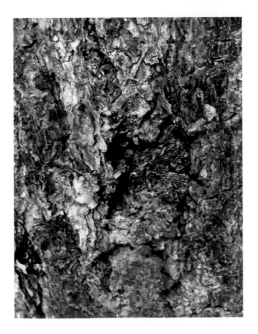

The bark is rough with a patch-work pattern full of fissures and breaks. If the tree has been damaged, we may see some of the sap oozing out, forming a resinous scab with its oily aroma.

sap can imbue the senses, evoking an impression of warmth and purification (and perhaps memories of household cleaning with pine oil).

When we awaken our own soul forces, we can then comprehend Nature as being formed by processes, rather than a mere collection of objects perceived by a mechanical consciousness. These processes are called the "formative forces" of Nature[40]. They belong to the etheric life realm and bestow life and form in the physical world.

In the pine, we experience these forces as the upward, light-seeking forces, especially the cleansing warmth embodied in the aromatic oils found in the leaves and sap. We gain an impression of the stature of the pine, constantly growing upward to the light. We can also appreciate the contrast between the light and dark poles of the plant: the dark earth with a heavy mat of dead needles around the tree, which discourages other plant life, and the somber green leaves that remain throughout the winter. At the same time, the pine is full of light, especially as we note its silica-rich leaves sparkling in the sun.

Recognition of archetypal or primal phenomena: The next step of research involves an appraisal of the organizing principles that provide further context for our experiences and observations. This differs from conventional scientific abstractions about general laws derived from data collection. For example, genetically-based botanists group plants according to the commonalities in their microscopic DNA structure. Bortoff calls this approach "unity in multiplicity."[41] He argues that the participatory science model of "multiplicity in unity," is a more living encounter. The organizing principle must be perceived in the phenomena itself. If this unifying archetype is accurately perceived, it can then be found in a variety of individual expressions. For example, the linear quality of

the conifers is expressed in various ways in the trunks, tap roots and needle-like leaves. It also finds diverse expression in the redwood, pine, spruce, fir, and other conifer species. If we compare and contrast the conifers with horizontally oriented branches of deciduous trees, this primary difference is even more noteworthy.

Moral imagination: The goal of participatory science is to deepen our appreciation of all living things in Nature, so that we experience the qualities that emanate from them. This process is not instantaneous. It may involve artistic study, collection of further data, a group exchange with others involved in the same research, and the continual interplay of our own meditations and observations. Our devotion to this process leads us to what Goethe called the unique "gesture," or essential inner quality of what is expressed. Ultimately, the ability to embrace such qualities as living experiences in our souls, leads to a moral awakening.

As we visit the pine again and again, we feel its particular radiance. We sense a distinct energetic shift in our own being, a vertical alignment that orients itself to the upward streaming of light. A quality of warmth enters into us that dissipates our attachment to the past. If we are prone to a saturnine or melancholic mood of soul, we can feel the purifying, uplifting quality of light in the pine as a healing balm. From such insights we can begin to understand Dr. Bach's indications for soul healing with the Pine flower essence. It helps to release and cleanse brooding melancholia. It is especially beneficial for one who becomes over-attached to past mistakes or excessive self-blame. The Pine flower essence brings warmth and uplifting light into the soul, transforming melancholia. It provides an impetus to the soul to accept the lessons of previous experience and move toward the future with self-confidence.[42]

If we want to achieve a living understanding of Nature, we must become as mobile and flexible as Nature herself.

— Johann von Goethe

For I have learned
To look on nature, not as in the hour
Of thoughtless youth; but hearing oftentimes
The still, sad music of humanity,
Nor harsh nor grating, though of ample power
To chasten and subdue. And I have felt
A presence that disturbs me with the joy
Of elevated thoughts; a sense sublime
Of something far more deeply interfused,
Whose dwelling is the light of setting suns,
And the round ocean and the living air,
And the blue sky, and in the mind of man;
A motion and a spirit, that impels
All thinking things, all objects of all thought,
And rolls through all things.
Therefore am I still
A lover of the meadows and the woods,
And mountains; and of all that we behold
From this green earth; of all the mighty world
Of eye, and ear, both what they half create,
And what perceive; well pleased to recognise
In nature and the language of the sense,
The anchor of my purest thoughts, the nurse,
The guide, the guardian of my heart, and soul
Of all my moral being.

William Wordsworth from "Tintern Abbey"

End Notes

1. *Health Week* (Program 408), PBS Broadcast, December 8, 2000.

2. See the article by Dr. Jeffrey Cram on page 89 of this issue.

3. Benveniste, J.,"Human basophil degranulation triggered by very dilute antiserum against IgE," *Nature,* 333: 816-818, 1988.
Plasterk, Ronald H.A., et al; "Explanation of Benveniste," *Nature,* 334:285, 1988.
Maddox, John; "'High-Dilution Experiments a Delusion," *Nature,* 334: 287, 1988. Written in conjunction with J. Randi and W.W. Stewart, with a reply by J. Benveniste.

4. Two early works: Bohm, David, *Wholeness and the Implicate Order,* Routeledge & Kegan Paul, Ltd., London, 1980 and
Capra, Fritjof, *The Tao of Physics,* Shambala Publications, Boston, MA, 1975.

5. See Gerber, Richard, MD, *Vibrational Medicine,* Bear & Company, Rochester, VT, 2001, or the International Society for the Subtle Energies and Energy Medicine, 11005 Ralston Road, Suite 100D, Arvada, CO, 80004, 303-425-4625, www.issseem.org.

6. Cram, J.R. , "A psychological and metaphysical study of Dr. Edward Bach's flower essence stress formula," *Subtle Energies and Energy Medicine Journal,* 2000. and Cram, J. R., "Effects of two flower essences on high intensity environmental stimulation and EMF," *Subtle Energies and Energy Medicine Journal,* 2002.
These studies are also available at www.flowersociety.org.

7. See article on page 89 of this journal.

8. See article on page 107 of this journal.

9. Kaminski, Patricia, *Flowers that Heal,* Gill and Macmillan, Dublin, Ireland, 1998, and her article starting on page 6 of this journal.

10. Also known as "Heisenberg's Indeterminacy Principle." See Bohm, David, *Wholeness and the Implicate Order,* Routeledge & Kegan Paul, Boston, 1982, pp. 69-70.

11. See Steiner, Rudolf, *An Outline of Esoteric Science,* SteinerBooks, Great Barrington, MA, 1997, for a discussion of one view of the evolution of human consciousness.

12. Cayce, Evans, *Edgar Cayce on Atlantis,* Warner Books, New York, 1968.

13. Steiner, Rudolf, *Cosmic Memory,* Garber Books, Blauvelt, NY, 1990.

14. See Morton, A.G., *History of Botanical Science,* Academic Press, London, 1981. Much of the historical information that follows is taken from this source.

15. Two of his better known works are *Systema naturae* (1735) and *Species plantarum,* (1753).

16. Cronquist, Arthur. *The evolution and classification of flowering plants,* Houghton Mifflin, Boston, 1988. Other commonly used systems are those of Armen Takhtajan, *Diversity and Classification of Flowering Plants,* Columbia University Press, New York, 1997.
Thorne, Robert, "Classification and Geography of Flowering Plants," *Botanical Review,* 58: 225-348, New York Botanical Garden, New York, 1992.

17. Darwin, Charles, *The Origin of Species,* 1859.

18. Watson, James D. with Andrew Berry, *DNA: The Secret of Life*, Random House, New York, 2003.

19. Cronquist, Takhtajan, Dahlgren and Thorne (see prior note).

20. Angiosperm Phylogeny Group, "An Ordinal Classification for the Families of Flowering Plants," *Annals of the Missouri Botanical Garden,* 85: 531-553, 1998, St. Louis, Missouri.

21. http://ucjeps.berkeley.edu/bryolab/GPphylo/

22. http://ucjeps.berkeley.edu/bryolab/deepgene/

23. http://www.natureinstitute.org

24. Holdrege, Craig, *Genetics and the Manipulation of Life: The Forgotten Factor of Context,* Lindisfarne Press, Hudson, NY, 1996.

25. Holdrege, Craig and Wirz, Johannes, "Life Beyond Genes: Reflections on the Human Genome Project," *In Context #5,* Spring 2001, pp. 14-19.

26. Bortoff, Henri. *The Wholeness of Nature, Goethe's Way toward a Science of Conscious Participation in Nature,* Lindisfarne Press, Hudson, NY, 1996.

27. See Allen, Paul Marshall, ed., *A Christian Rosenkreutz Anthology,* Garber Books, Blauvelt, NY, 2000, and
Steiner, Rudolf, *Christian Rosenkreutz: The Mystery, Teaching and Mission of a Master,* Rudolf Steiner Press, London, 2002.

28. Jocabi, Jolande, ed. *Paracelsus, Selected Writings,* Princeton University Press, Princeton, NJ, 1951, 1995.

29. Gerard, John, *The Herbal: Or, General History of Plants,* Dover Publications, New York, NY, 1975.

30. Culpeper, Nicholas, *Culpeper's Complete Herbal and English Physician,* Meyerbooks, Glenwood, Illinois, 1987.

31. A popular biography of Kepler is Caspar, Max, et. al, *Kepler,* Dover Publications, New York, NY, 1993. Also see Koestler, Arthur, *The Sleepwalkers,* Peregrine Books, London, 1988.

32. Miller, Douglas, ed. and trans., *Goethe: The Collected Works, Volume 12: Scientific Studies,* Princeton University Press, Princeton, NJ, 1995.
Botanical drawing is from Goethe's *Metamorphosis of Plants,* as reprinted in *Goethe's Botanical Writings,* tr. by Bertha Mueller, Ox Bow Press, Woodbridge, CT 1989, p.47.
Goethe's "Nature," poem excerpt from *Aphorisms,* 1869, translated by T.H. Huxley.
Highlighted quotations from
Goethe, Johann *Goethe's Botanical Writings,* tr. by Bertha Mueller, Ox Bow Press, Woodbridge, CT 1989.
Goethe, Johann, *Goethe's World View, Ungar Publishing Company, New York, NY, 1958.*

33. Darwin, Charles, *Origin of Species,* Gramercy, New York, NY, 1979 (originally published 1859).

34. Steiner, Rudolf, *Nature's Open Secret: Introductions to Goethe's Scientific Writings,* Anthroposophic Press, Great Barrington, MA, 2000. This book contains Steiner's early commentary on Goethe's scientific studies.

35. Adams, George, and Whicher, Olive, *The Plant Between Sun and Earth,* Rudolf Steiner Press, London, 1980.

36. Edwards, Lawrence, *The Vortex of Life,* Floris Books, Edinburgh, Scotland, 1993.

37. Grohmann, Gerbert, *The Plant, Vols. 1 & 2,* Biodynamic Literature, Kimberton, PA, 1989.

38. Pelikan, Wilhelm, *Healing Plants: Insights through Spiritual Science, Volume 1,* Mercury Press, Spring Valley, NY 1997.

39. Goethe, Johann, *Metamorphosis of Plants,* found in *Goethe: The Collected Works, Volume 12, Scientific Studies,* edited and translated by Douglas Miller, Princeton University Press, Princeton, NJ, 1995.

40. For an excellent example of nature observation that is cognizant of such forces, see von Romunde, *About Formative Forces in the Plant World,* translated and published by Jannebeth Röell, Cortlandt Manor, New York, 2001.

41. Bortoff, *op. cit.* pp. 82-89.

42. For another discussion of the qualities of the Pine essence in relationship to the botany of the Pine tree, see Barnard, Julian, *Bach Flower Remedies: Form & Function,* Lindisfarne Books, Great Barrington, MA, 2004, pages 258-263. Barnard's book is an excellent application of the methods of participatory science to an understanding of Dr. Bach's flower essences. Also see the discussion of the Rose and Sunflower families in Patricia Kaminski's article, pages 19-29 of this journal.

The Medical Practice of Dr. Audun Myskja in Norway

Healing the Body, Transforming the Soul

by Richard Katz

Dr. Audun Myskja is a medical doctor whose life path and inner experience resembles Dr. Edward Bach. He has learned that true healing involves the transformation of the soul, not merely the repair of the body. Like Dr. Bach, his own healing journey took him through the gates of illness into a life of service dedicated to healing others. He is a renowned author, teacher, and researcher in Norway who champions holistic therapies and educates mainstream medical practitioners. His work with music therapy for the elderly was awarded recognition by the Norwegian Medical Association in 1998 and 2002. His first flower essence book, **Blomstermedisin til vekst og helbredelse (Flower Essences for Growth and Healing)**[1] is a recommended text in the advanced education for nurses and social workers at Hogskolen i Oslo (the regional University in the Oslo region). It is a three-hundred page hardbound book, replete with in-depth case studies for each of Dr. Bach's flower essences.

A Connection with Nature

Born in 1953, in Trondheim, Norway, Dr. Myskja describes his youth as "turbulent" and "marked by illness." He found strength and solace in Nature by opening to the healing qualities of plants: "I discovered that specific species of flowers and trees seemed to have different effects on me: in a certain type of turmoil, mountain birches would have a soothing effect that I could never get from contacting other trees. I started being interested in herbal medicine, and would notice that **Yarrow** seemed to give a specific protection when I felt vulnerable, enabling me to keep my balance in a

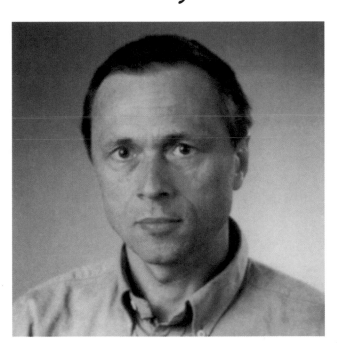

city environment, while **Iris** would strengthen inspiration when I felt dull."

A Calling to be a Healer

At the age of 21, a friend gave him Dr. Bach's *Heal Thyself.* Dr. Bach's treatise gave voice to his own experiences and yearnings. During this time, he underwent what he calls "an Edward Bach-like experience." He describes his illness worsening until it, "culminated in a near-death experience that gave me my life's calling: to become a doctor and work to integrate spiritual and natural dimensions in medical practice." After volunteer work in several countries, and university studies in philosophy, psychology and comparative religions, Myskja began his medical studies in 1975 in Bergen, Norway. He did his clinical training in Trondheim, Norway, receiving his medical degree in 1981. During his medical studies, he was already practicing as a naturopath. "Doing what I was meant to do filled my life to such an extent that I found myself having no time for illness," he reflected. "I do not intend this to sound facile, but this is actually what happened: it was as if the contact with others' suffering consumed my own. From the experience of being a miserable youth, I have basically been a happy adult (assisted by the flower essences)."

Music as Therapy

Devoted to music from the time of his youth, Dr. Myskja sang and wrote songs, and played guitar and harmonica, the latter on a professional level. Music became a healing modality for him after studies in toning from Anne Parks[2], and meditation and energy studies with Bob Moore[3]. During the 1980's, he developed music therapy with his patients to address lethargy, depression and anxiety, with seminars integrating meditation, toning, voice work and music as self-healing tools. During the 1990's, Dr. Myskja designed music therapy for use in health services, particularly in geriatrics and palliative care. While medical director of Hospice Lovisenberg in Oslo (1998-99), his first book *Den Musiske Medisin (Musical Medicine)*[4] was published. He now develops music therapy programs for a number of nursing homes in Norway, trains medical and dental students in music therapy, and is conducting scientific research to document the healing effects of music therapy in the elderly population.

A Phenomenological Approach to Flower Essence Therapy

Since 1976, Dr. Myskja has included flower essence therapy in his clinical practice, including Dr. Bach's original remedies as well as new essences. At least 10-20 of his patients daily receive flower essence therapy as part of their healing program. Dr. Myskja has been teaching flower essence therapy since 1989, reaching many Norwegian naturopaths and holistic practitioners. Since the publication of *Blomstermedisin til vekst og helbredelse* in 2000, flower essence therapy has attracted the attention of mainstream medical professionals.

Dr. Myskja describes his therapeutic approach as "phenomenological," taking into account flower essence published research, information given by the patient, body language, and energetic expression. All of these phenomena form a fuller gestalt, leading to the selection of appropriate flower

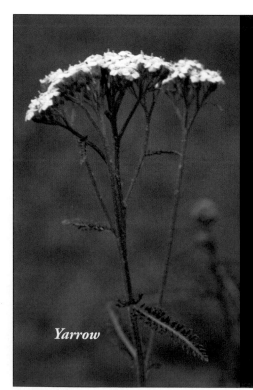

Yarrow

Yarrow seemed to give a specific protection when I felt vulnerable, enabling me to keep my balance in a city environment, while Iris would strengthen inspiration when I felt dull.

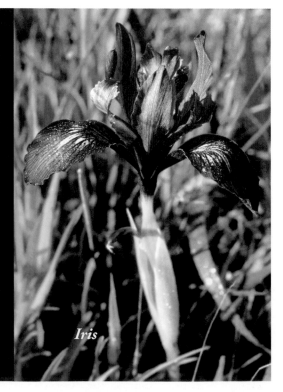

Iris

essences for each individual client. Dr. Myskja previously selected remedies via pendulum and kinesiology, but has reached the conclusion that this method can be problematic, leading to "spiritual laziness" and avoidance of the "necessary relationship with the person."

Groundbreaking Case: Treating Severe Eczema with Flower Essences

Flower essence therapy achieved greater public awareness in 2001 when Norway's largest weekly family magazine *Hjemmet*, read by over one quarter of Norway's population, published an article about one of Dr. Myskja's cases.[5] This case involved a young girl who developed severe eczema and asthma after a protracted birth. Treated in hospital, by specialists in pediatrics and allergies, she was prescribed cortisone in large doses. Her mother was concerned about the adverse effects of cortisone, and attempted alternative measures such herbal medicine, homeopathy, and reflexology. None of these modalities were effective until Dr. Myskja developed an intensive flower essence therapy program, utilizing **Rescue Remedy cream, Rock Rose, Crab Apple, Aspen, Walnut, and Star of Bethlehem,** supplemented by daily reflexology and massage by the mother. The essences addressed the child's hypersensitivity and originating birth trauma, as well as the effects of her mother's anxiety and stress after her birth. Within three months, the child's eczema was barely visible and did not produce irritation and itching. Her mother was highly impressed by the success of this natural approach, after expensive and cumbersome treatments with potential side-effects had failed to help her daughter. She reported her case to *Hjemmet* magazine, and the article was widely read throughout Scandinavia.

While flower essence therapy in Norway has grown steadily, it remains predominant among natural health practitioners. Only 7% of Norwegian doctors are open to alternative medicine (with only 1% actively involved) compared to 30% in Denmark and Bavaria (southern Germany). With the emphasis on "evidence-based medicine," credible research in flower essence therapy is crucial. Dr. Myskja feels the situation will change when enough health professionals:

☆ have personal experience with the positive effects of flower essences,

☆ meet enough colleagues who have documented their successful cases,

☆ encounter patients who have clearly benefited from flower essences,

☆ have access to professional literature that specifically addresses flower essence phenomena.

Developing Professional Flower Essence Research

Given his goal of reaching skeptical medical professionals with the benefits of flower essence therapy, Myskja is concerned about a lack of interest in quality control or evaluation procedures in the flower essence community. He describes a prevalent attitude as "I am a humble, egoless, pure channel of God, therefore no one can in any way question my methods or decisions. Thus, by definition, I am always right." This emphasis on subjective "inward guidance" often obscures the need for objective observation and conscious methods of evaluation.

Dr. Myskja has been impressed with the research objectives of the ***Flower Essence Society***. He regards Dr. Jeffrey Cram's double-blind studies with stress to be among the most persuasive when he is asked by colleagues for scientific backing for flower essences. He comments that randomized double-blind studies are the most persuasive with the medical profession, but that clinical studies are more likely to have successful outcomes, given the importance of individualized treatment and personal relationship in flower essence therapy.

Treating the Elderly

Dr. Myskja intends to collaborate with the Flower Essence Society and other institutes to develop research protocols for elderly populations. He believes there is an urgent need for alternatives to standard treatments for the elderly, particularly for agitation and depression. He comments, "It has been documented[6] that drugs for agitation don't work (beyond placebo level) in therapeutic doses with the elderly. The drugs have to be given in larger doses (up to 4 or 5 times therapeutic dose) to reduce agitation significantly. In reducing agitation, one may then also reduce vitality and well-being. It is therefore important to combine pharmaceutical treatment with non-pharmacological measures. Music has been shown to be effective. I would like to do serious research on flower essences in this context, since I have seen them work in single cases."

A solid foundation for flower essence research has been established through Dr. Myskja's research in music therapy and extensive contacts with nursing homes. For example, he has collaborated with the five nursing homes of the Kirkens Bymisjon (Inner City Mission) in Oslo. This 150-year old charitable organization seeks life-affirming therapies for approximately 500 elderly, infirm and incurable patients.

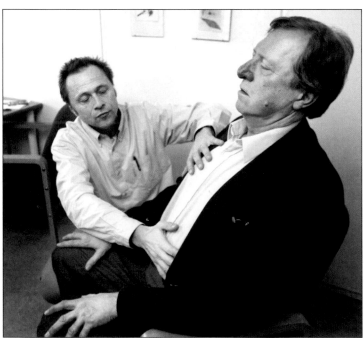

Health practitioners interested in a clinical research program using flower essences with elderly clients, are invited to contact the **Flower Essence Society** (research@flowersociety.org) or Dr. Myskja at info@livshjelp.no.

Current Activities

Audun Myskja lives with his family in Oppegaard, a suburb south of Oslo, 20 minutes away by car or train. His house is at the edge of a forest — "as quiet as it gets this near Oslo." His wife Reidun is an experienced homeopath, reflexologist, counselor and specialist in natural products. His children, Maria Ray, Rafael and Sakarias, ages 18, 14 and 11, still live at home.

Together with his wife Reidun, Dr. Myskja runs the "Senter for Livshjelp" (Tools for Healing) nearby in Ski, a clinic where he has a small practice and conducts workshops in flower essence therapy, toning, meditation and self-healing. He has made several musical recordings, is a prolific lecturer and writer, especially on music in medicine. He is currently leading the following projects:

☆ Music as an aid in palliative care in nursing homes — 3-year project in Oslo, 2002-4,

☆ Rhythm as an aid for Parkinson's Disease patients — 3-year project nationwide, 2003-5,

☆ Music as an aid in palliative care in nursing homes — 3-year research doctorate project in Bergen, 2004-6.

Dr. Myskja treats a 57-year old cancer patient with severe lymphoma. He is a scientist at the University of Oslo and was treated with flower essences while undergoing chemotherapy. Dr. Myskja believes his successful chemotherapy — his tumors have regressed — was aided by the flower essences he utilized. This picture is from a full page article in Norway's most influential newspaper Aftenposten *concerning Dr. Myskja's work with complementary treatments, published February 10, 2004.*

Three Typical Cases Reported by Dr. Myskja

A Young Executive Recovers from Fatigue and Hair Loss

Arne was a dynamic executive in his early forties, who joined a high paced computer software firm. He worked long hours six days a week, with irregular sleep and exercise. The intensity of his experience was satisfying until his firm experienced a financial slump. He started to feel pressure, as optimism gave way to negative messages, and the results were no longer proportionate with the output. His pace of work led to a traumatic break in a long-term personal relationship that he had taken for granted.

Gradually, Arne developed lethargy verging on depression, with chronic symptoms following influenza. He consulted his medical doctor and was diagnosed with post-viral fatigue. Paradoxically, Arne originally contacted me for another problem: he had always had a thick head of hair, like other men in his family, but now his hair was visibly thinning. This made him panic, and he sought my help to see if there were natural remedies to counteract this development.

It was obvious that Arne had been under chronic stress for some time, and exhibited signs of an ongoing alarm reaction in body and mind. Blood tests had been normal, and I felt that he needed stress management. I taught him relaxation exercises and guided imagery in music, including exercises and massage instructions for tight scalp and neck tissue. I used the following flower essences: **Cotton** for mental vitality, **Lemon** for cleansing (internal use and topical doses for the scalp), **Nasturtium** for his mental strain and arid intellectual life, **Self-Heal** to strengthen his over-all healing capacity and **Ylang Ylang** essential oil as a general stress-reducing tonic. I encouraged him to spend at least 30-60 minutes in Nature each day, and to engage in breathing exercises.

When Arne returned for the next consultation, he reported a difference, which he described as feeling "a growing plant within him." He also reported feeling slight tinges of joy breaking through his lethargy and depression. At the next consultation, he reported excitedly, "I can feel new hair coming up in my bald spots!" I explained this was possible in his case, since he had a thick scalp that was not genetically prone to baldness. Prolonged stress with scalp constriction was probably the main culprit in his hair loss.

Arne's basic constitutional remedy was **Vervain**, a remedy for intense drive and enthusiasm. I included this core remedy with the other essences in his formula. He learned to curb his incessant outward drive and find an anchor of calm in situations that previously produced a stress spiral. Arne experienced a full recovery within half a year, prompted by his growing self-awareness and the recognition that he needed to find a balance between his inner motivation and the outer situation.

Comments on this case: I feel certain that the recovery of Arne's head hair and the healing from chronic fatigue and depression would have been impossible without flower essences. Yet, flower essences alone did not bring about the healing. The essences act basically as "inner enzymes" to facilitate growth and healing processes. In children and animals, they can be given as a simple measure, while in adults with symptoms of complex origin, they often need to be a part of a many-faceted regime, tailor-made for the individual's needs. One must direct the flower essences not only to the external symptoms, but also to an understanding of deeper issues involving the genesis, role and function of illness in the person's life. My successful cases are often based on a combination of an inner willingness to change, lifestyle/situation and attitudinal shifts, mental/spiritual and physical exercises tailored to the individual, flower essences and other natural therapies, supplemented with specific physical exercises, music and awareness programs.

Treating Extreme Environmental Sensitivity in a Young Woman

Flower essences produced dramatic results with Carla, a young woman in her early thirties who was a rebel in a prominent family with bourgeois values. She revolted, joined an oppositional culture, and traveled around Europe, meeting like-minded persons. Along the way, she experimented with drugs and sexuality and neglected regular meals and sleep. When she returned to Norway, she married and soon became pregnant. However, the strain of her previous lifestyle had taken its toll, and she had a difficult pregnancy, bedridden with back and pelvic pain most of the time.

After the baby's birth, she suffered from extreme fatigue, with oversensitivity to electro-magnetic fields. She was unable to work since nearly all jobs involved computers or related technology, and manual work was too demanding. Carla received a disability pension, and devoted most of her time to the basic tasks of life, including dressing and eating. Despite consultation with various therapists and medical doctors, antidepressants and megadoses of vitamins and minerals only worsened her condition. Body therapies were too intense for her sensitive condition and resulted in extreme reactions.

When I first consulted with Carla, she felt drained of energy, with no hope of recovery. I gave her polarity exercises to balance and build up her vital field, and taught her how to make contact with large trees, such as oak and elm, for one-half hour each day. I gave her **Gorse** and **Olive** flower essences for her hopelessness and lethargy. I chose **Cerato** as her constitutional remedy — to heal her deep lack of trust in her own spiritual core and her feeling of being an "outsider" in her family system. I supplemented with **Yarrow** for hypersensitivity to electromagnetic fields, and **Morning Glory** as a tonic to heal the effects of her earlier excessive lifestyle. Carla followed my regime faithfully, and engaged in Nature meditations to draw on the reservoir of natural healing impulses in the surrounding countryside and sea coast.

When Carla returned in one month, I noticed that she seemed lighter and more erect. After the second month, she described a new strength rising, like "sap in spring." Her motivation grew as she perceived results. She developed the strength to go out in Nature and seek healing. Her self-respect increased by engaging her complete attention in her healing program. Carla recovered, with the aid of flower essences as indispensable catalysts. As she herself says: "**I could feel the flower drops working as a gradual change in my perception and my attitudes. In fact, it was as if the flower essences enabled me to change.**"

Comments on the case: In my experience, changing chronic conditions has to do with changing a vicious cycle, one that is imprinted physiologically in neuro-hormonal circuits and receptor systems, and psychologically in lack of self-esteem and motivation.

> I chose Cerato as her constitutional remedy — to heal her deep lack of trust in her own spiritual core and her feeling of being an "outsider" in her family system.

Cerato

An Artist Encounters Life with Flower Essences instead of Psychiatric Drugs

Lina is an artist in her late thirties who experienced serious mental imbalances during adolescence. At the time of her treatment from me, she had been through two major psychotic episodes, one after childbirth, the other after a meditation seminar. Though I do not generally work as a psychiatric doctor, I became aware of a hidden potential in Lina for understanding interior states of soul consciousness. She enrolled in my seminars, and responded well to flower essences, including **Clematis** (her constitutional remedy), **Cherry Plum, Walnut, Wild Oat and Rock Rose.** She could feel a distinct response to each dose of this combination — helping her to experience normalcy, drive and direction in life.

Lina's experience of Clematis was especially vivid, addressing the inner split between mind and body, and drawing them closer together. She started expressing her own recognition of finer levels of consciousness. At first, her words were awkward,

Lina's experience of Clematis was especially vivid, addressing the inner split between mind and body, and drawing them closer together.

Clematis

as she attempted to express inner experiences, but gradually she became more articulate, evidencing an inner authority that made people listen. She developed a gift for reaching people on the fringes of society and helping them return to life, just as she herself had been helped.

Lina now consults with difficult pupils in schools, participates in conferences on human consciousness, and dialogues with prominent scientists and philosophers. Lina has become a remarkable and original flower essence practitioner, well versed in several therapeutic systems, and researching Norwegian flower essences.

Comments on this case: This is one of my most striking cases. I have followed Lina for over a decade, and know for sure that she would have been a psychiatric patient on drugs, with a disability pension, had she not discovered the flower essences and the right self-development tools at a crucial crossroads in her life. Intense psychiatric drugs and hospitalization would have prevented the gradual soul healing she has experienced over the last decade. My dream is that other sensitive souls, locked in a psychic dream world that avoids the challenging conditions of earth life, can be helped with flower essence therapy, guidance, and inner work.

End Notes

[1] *Blomstermedisin til vekst og helbredelse,* Oslo, Norway: Noras Ark, 2000.

[2] An American healer (unpublished) who was Dr. Myskja's teacher while she lived in Europe 1976-78. He describes her as "the most formative influence in my grown years, after my family and vocation."

[3] Irish-born spiritual teacher (unpublished), clairvoyant, scientifically trained, lived in Ringkøbing, Denmark, in the period 1978-1998. Dr. Myskja took part in his workshops several weekends/weeks a year until he retired.

[4] *Hjemmet,* 43/2001: Oslo; Hjemmet Mortensen AS.

[5] *Den musiske medisin,* Oslo: Grøndahl Dreyer, 1999.

[6] Teri L, Logsdon RG, Peskind E, Raskind M, Weiner MF, Tractenberg RE, Foster NL, Schneider LS, Sano M, Whitehouse P, Tariot P, Mellow AM, Auchus AP, Grundman M, Thomas RG, Schafer K, Thal LJ. Treatment of agitation in AD: a randomized, placebo-controlled clinical trial. *Neurology.* 2000 Nov 14;55(9):1247-8. University of Washington, Department of Psycho-social and Community Health, Seattle 98195-7263, USA. Lteri@u.washington.edu.

Healing Fear & Finding Love
Flower Therapy for Disadvantaged Children in Campinas, Brazil
by Rosana Souto Sobral Vieira

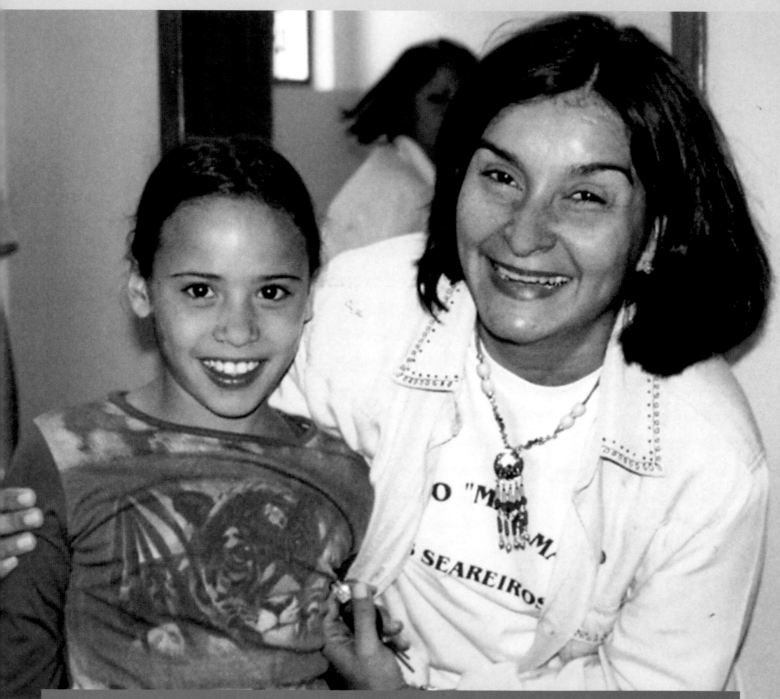

When working with disadvantaged children ... we are called to do our deepest and most compassionate work. The time cannot be wasted, for there may be only a single chance to make a difference in their lives.

Núcleo Mãe Maria is a social institution maintained by Os Seareiros, a religious charity that organizes professional volunteer teams of health practitioners and educators to serve the needs of about 350 families in the Vila Brandina community of Campinas, Brazil. This region is a major drug center of the city, marked by violence as well as poverty. Children grow up in an atmosphere of great terror. Almost every child we help has witnessed murder and other extreme brutality. On the other hand, Vila Brandina is also the home of decent poor people who work hard, and must leave their children with either relatives or alone in the home while at work.

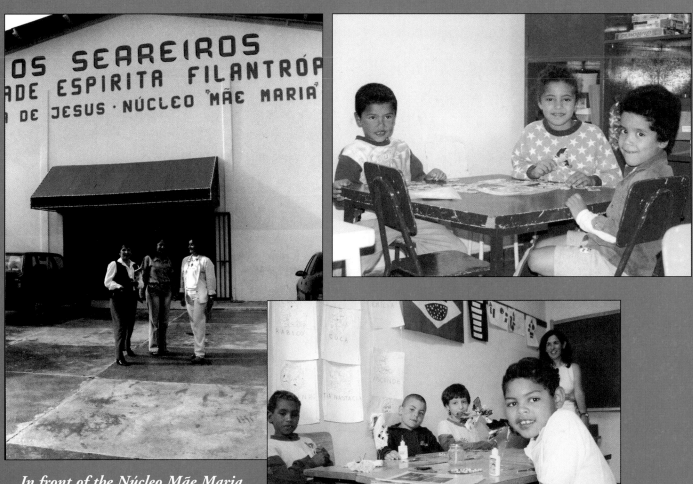

In front of the Núcleo Mãe Maria office (left to right): Teresa Diegues, flower essence therapist; Leonor C. Moussali, the institution's Educational Coordinator and General Manager; Rosana Vieira, the founder and Coordinator of Flower Therapy at Núcleo Mãe Maria

Classrooms at the Núcleo Mãe Maria

The Child's Soul Identity — Not Answers but Questions

During my years of practice at Núcleo Mãe Maria, I have gathered clear evidence that learning disorders are usually the final manifestation of early birth traumas, including rejection, abandonment, violence, sexual abuse and fear, as well as nutritional and hereditary factors. Sometimes a single bottle of the remedies has been enough to change the life perspective of a child in dramatic ways.

We have found that it is important to have a team of professionals, each one reporting to another and working for a common result. Our educational supervisor, who is able to view the progress of the children from another vantage point, describes the unique role of the flower essences as helping the child to find a center, or core identity for encountering life. This deeper identity of the child must always be considered, for we cannot simply change the outer behavior. It is impossible to help the children of Núcleo Mãe Maria without addressing their emotional past. These wounds affect their current behavior as well as their future potential.

I can only approach my work — not by having answers — but by asking questions. For instance, when I work with emotionally distant, absent-minded, or ungrounded children, I always ask myself: "What makes them refuse to be here? Why are they not grounded, or connected with their bodies?" I realize that the pain of being in their bodies is so great. I know that I cannot bring them fully to earth without providing tools to face their reality. When working with disadvantaged children, there are many "whats" and "whys" to answer. We are called to do our deepest and most compassionate work. The time cannot be wasted, for there may be only a single chance to make a difference in their lives.

Flower Essence Formulating: Creating "Attunement"

I believe that flower essence therapy is a healing modality that can be understood scientifically, but also has to be practiced artistically. I have a musical background, and every time I make a formula it seems to me that I am creating a song. It is a healing structure that literally brings "attunement" by helping the client to hear the "tune" or musical harmony that resonates within the soul, resolving dissonances that stand in the way. Like music, the healing effects of flower essences are rhythmic, and we are challenged to create the necessary patterns and timing so that each client can "hear" and respond to the composition.

Working with flower essence formulas has also allowed me to broaden my work at Núcleo Mãe Maria. Most of my healing work with the children is conducted on an individual basis. However, it is not possible to give specialized attention to every child, especially as our work has increased with more children every year. Therefore, I also consult with the teachers to design more general prescriptions for the classroom. These formulas are structured according to the main needs of each classroom. The applications may be standard internal dosages, but also include misting formulas for the environment of the classroom at least twice during the learning period. The teachers report this method is surprisingly effective, helping the concentration and general behavior of the students.

A dance performance by the students of Núcleo Mãe Maria.

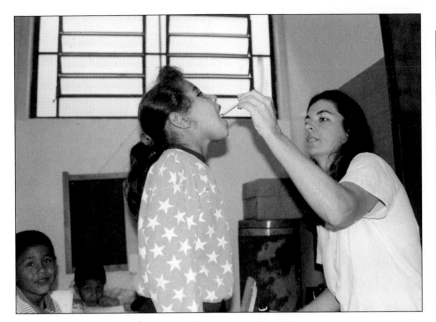

Flower essences are administered to the
children during class sessions.

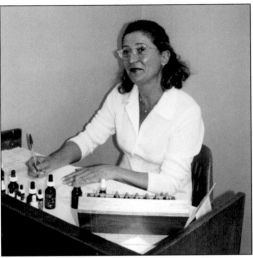

A volunteer at the Núcleo Mãe Maria.

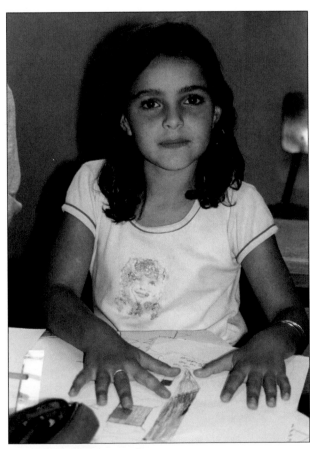

Art is an important part of the children's
program at Núcleo Mãe Maria.
Drawings from the students show many
flower and nature themes.

I believe that flower essence therapy is a healing modality that can be understood scientifically, but also has to be practiced artistically. I have a musical background, and every time I make a formula it seems to me that I am creating a song.

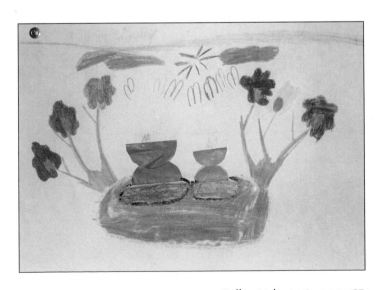

Providing Nurturing Forces for Young Children

Children who attend kindergarten (6 years of age) are now receiving flower essences early. The main strategy of my flower essence formulas is to help each child feel emotionally safe and receptive to learning. **Mariposa Lily** is a foundational remedy to provide nurturing and supportive forces and to heal disruptions in the mother-child bond. Other major essences that are frequently used include **Mimulus** (insecurity, shyness or a fearful response to common life situations), **Chestnut Bud** (to instill rhythms and patterns for learning, especially movement, perception and coordination), **Honeysuckle** (to enter a new life phase, to leave behind old memories or insecurities) and **Clematis** (to be present and alert and come more fully into the body).

Older Children — Restoring Dignity and Opening the Heart

Some of the older children are already involved in drug use and sexual behavior. Sometimes the whole family is involved in these activities and it is an extremely delicate situation to address. These children are more hardened or defended, and so we must start with very specific situations. The resolution of these symptoms is a pathway for receiving further therapeutic help, and a chance for these children to begin to reflect on their lives.

Some of the major flower essences indicated in such cases include **Vine** (to soften the heart and curb aggressive tendencies),

Baby Blue Eyes (to address cynicism and emotional dryness), **Saguaro** (to respect teachers and other authority figures, and to develop responsibility), **Willow** (to resolve resentment and feelings of injustice), **Chamomile** (to provide calming and ease explosive tempers), **Holly** (to heal the heart's pain and develop unconditional love and trust), and **Cherry Plum** (for loss of nervous control). These remedies are administered as internal dosages and are also utilized in misting bottles for the classroom.

Many children are exposed to sexuality very early. Some are abused, while others are exploited for monetary reasons. Many are gripped by addictive patterns that provide an escape from the intensity of their lives. Some of the key remedies that I use to address these issues are **Easter Lily** (to cleanse aspects of fallen or hardened sexuality that is divorced from a spiritual identity), **Heather** (for intense pre-occupation with sexuality or addictive tendencies such as masturbation), **Echinacea** (for trauma and assault to the core identity of the child) and **Baby Blue Eyes** (to restore dignity, trust and confidence, especially in the case of sexual abuse).

Wild Oat has been of great help to all of these children. It opens new life pathways and helps the children consider their unique talents waiting to be developed.

> **Inasmuch as you did it to one of the least of these My brethren, you did it to Me.**
>
> **Matthew 25:40**

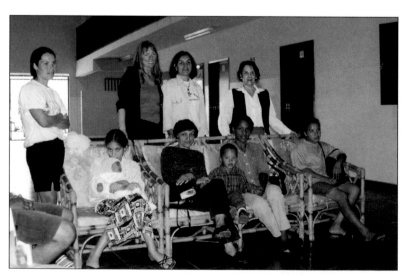

Rosana Vieira and others with Patricia Kaminski at the Núcleo Mãe Maria family outreach center.

The Greatest Need: Healing Fear and Finding Love

Fear is the greatest factor that influences the lives of all our children and inhibits their ability to learn. This fear is pervasive, throughout the community and neighborhoods, and affects the most intimate aspects of home life. Nightmares and bed-wetting, and other related syndromes are the most common result of this fear. Flower therapy is now widely known and respected in the village for its outstanding efficacy in resolving these problems. The primary flower essences used include **Mimulus** and **Rock Rose** (for fear and terror), **Cherry Plum** (for fear of losing control), **Chestnut Bud** (for repetitive behaviors and patterns), **Honeysuckle** (for regressive tendencies), **Saint John's Wort** (for protection during sleep), **Aspen** (for fear of what is unknown or new), and **Mariposa Lily** and **Chicory** (for nurturing and mothering).

Addressing Learning Disorders in a Soul Context

There are also many outstanding flower essences that can directly help the learning process such as **Clematis, Chestnut Bud, Impatiens, Shasta Daisy, Madia, Cerato, Larch, Cosmos, Rosemary,** and **Peppermint**. However, these flower essences won't be entirely effective unless we also address the deeper soul needs of each child. This requires not only a good knowledge of flower essences but, even more importantly, learning how to be alert and receptive to each child's unique feelings.

We are called to be open to feel each child and to respond with love in our hearts to their suffering. Needy children are not different from us, or from any other children — they seek to be loved and the flower essences can help nurture these soul impulses.

About Rosana Vieira

Rosana Souto Sobral Vieira has trained widely in the field of healing arts, including astrology and flower essence therapy. In 1990, she left her original career as a chemical engineer (State University of Rio de Janeiro, 1977) to dedicate her life to helping others. She is a flower essence therapist, teacher and a leader in establishing social service programs with flower essences.

Since 1998, she has been using flower essences to help children with severe learning disorders in her private practice and through her volunteer work at Núcleo Mãe Maria. Also, since 1998, she has been coordinating the social service center of the Brazilian Association of Flower Essences — ABRE-FLOR— in Campinas. Rosana Vieira founded the Instituto Cosmos de Terapia Floral (Cosmos Institute of Flower Therapy) in 1995, as a teaching and training center for flower essence therapy in the Campinas region of Brazil. She has attended Flower Essence Society classes and trainings in Brazil and California, and has completed her FES practitioner certification. She is authorized to teach the FES Practitioner Training and Certification program through her Cosmos Institute in Brazil, and is also authorized by Julian Barnard of Healing*herbs* to teach about Bach flowers in Brazil.

web site : www.cosmosinstituto.com.br
e-mail: rsvieira@sigmanet.com.br
tel/fax: +55 19 32334861

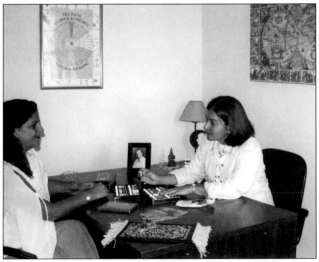

Rosana Vieira with a flower essence client.

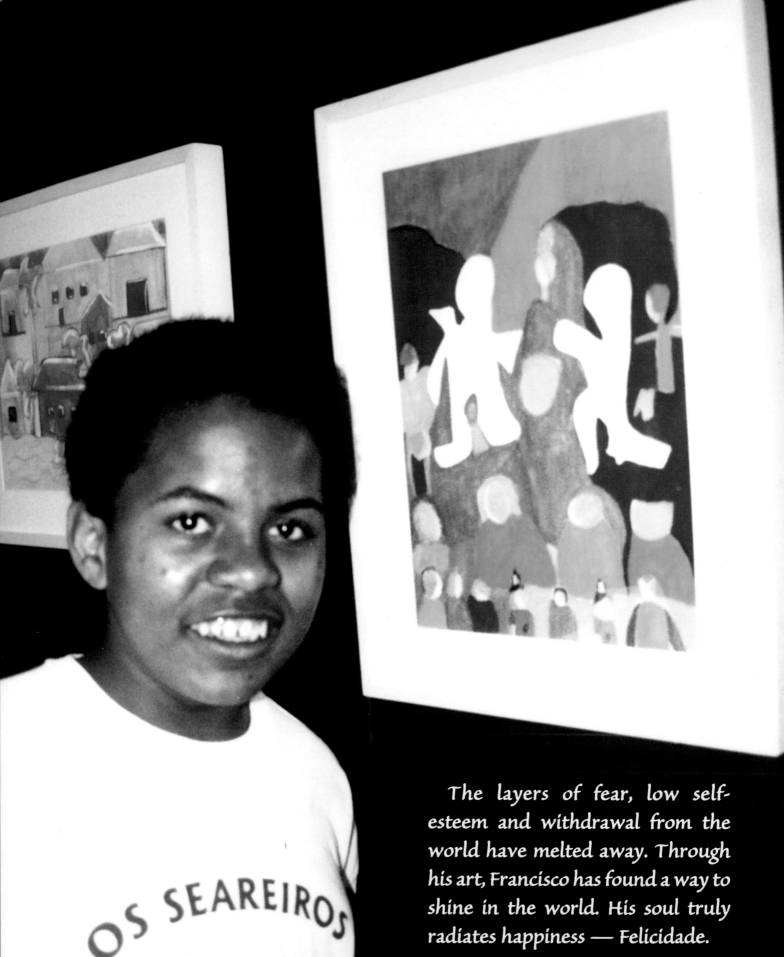

The layers of fear, low self-esteem and withdrawal from the world have melted away. Through his art, Francisco has found a way to shine in the world. His soul truly radiates happiness — Felicidade.

Felicidade

How the Flowers Helped Francisco Find a Happy Heart

a case study by Rosana Souto Sobral Vieira

A Violent Home Life and Severe Learning Problems

Francisco was one of my earliest clients. At the time when I first consulted with him, he was a boy of nearly 13 years of age with severe learning difficulties, hardly able to read or write. He suffered from continual nightmares and bed-wetting. Francisco's home life was very violent with an alcoholic father and a depressive mother. His father resorted to beating family members for the slightest reason.

When I first saw Francisco, it was following a traumatic fight with his father, in which he tried to protect his mother from being beaten. His physical appearance was stocky and strong, but unkempt. He was not socially present or embodied, and he was unexpressive. He answered all my questions with, "Don't know." I asked him to draw anything he would like. After a short period of reluctance, he drew a tiny boy in the middle of the page. This drawing showed me clearly how withdrawn he was from his body and soul. His self-portrait covered only a small portion of the large paper and it was composed of non-flowing blocks and rectangles. (See drawing below.)

My first strategy was to heal his emotional trauma and re-instill life force in his body and confidence in his soul. (At that time the range of flower essences available to the center was more limited. For cases similar to Francisco's, especially involving urinary disturbances, I now include **St. John's Wort** in my therapeutic approach.)

During the first two months the flower essences used were: **Clematis, Chestnut Bud, Mimulus, Rock Rose, Cherry Plum, Chicory, Scleranthus, Gentian, Crab Apple, Honeysuckle** and **Holly**. In addition to emotional support from the above remedies, a Learning Formula of **Rosemary, Shasta Daisy**, and **Peppermint** was also used.

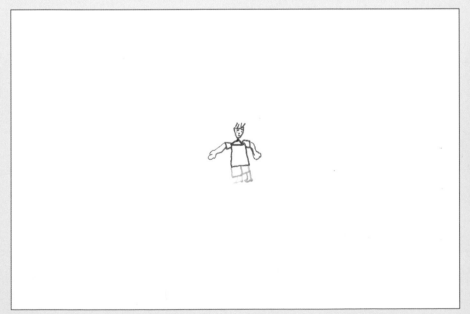

I asked him to draw anything he would like. After a short period of reluctance, he drew a tiny boy in the middle of the page. This drawing showed me clearly how withdrawn he was from his body and soul.

Dramatic Improvement

Francisco showed dramatic improvement in just one month. He was present, alert, and tried to answer my questions with sentences other than "Don't know." He was completely free from his former nightmares and bed-wetting episodes. Francisco was very impressed with the results and was very willing to continue treatment with me. He was so captivated by the flower medicines, that he wanted to draw a picture of a flower fairy. This picture is more expressive than his first one, with the arms opening to the world. However, a badge is still over the heart area. (See drawing below.)

In the third month, his mother consulted with me. She was very pleased to report that she also noticed the remarkable developments in Francisco, and she confirmed that his urinary disturbances remained completely resolved both at home and in school. One interesting note was that the teachers reported Francisco was no longer withdrawn and, in fact, was speaking too much in class, sometimes being very demanding of attention. These swings in soul mood with flower essence therapy are typical, as the soul seeks to establish a new balance. Also, Francisco had improved in his writing skills but still remained slow in reading.

The flower essences used for Francisco during this time were: **Clematis, Chestnut Bud, Mimulus, Holly, Cherry Plum, Rock Rose, Crab Apple, Chicory, Heather, Vervain, Cerato, Larch, Wild Oat** and **Blackberry.** The Learning Formula of **Rosemary, Shasta Daisy** and **Peppermint** was also continued.

Standing on Solid Earth

During the next month-and-a-half Francisco remained embodied and alert, although there were still some challenges in studying. Francisco had also gained weight and appeared more incarnated in his body. He conveyed great happiness about his flower essences and he expressed the wish to attend art classes. He drew another picture showing himself much bigger and more grounded. Very significantly, his soul is expressing a desire to receive and be connected with the forces of nature. He is standing on solid earth, surrounded by trees with the sun shining over him. These kinds of pictures, showing a relationship to nature in the soul, are a very typical development for children who are using flower essences. (See drawing on the next page.)

By the fourth meeting, the teachers reported changes in Francisco's social behavior. Previously, he had seemed numb in his interactions with others; then, he had become more sensitive, and showed feelings if he was provoked or was teased.

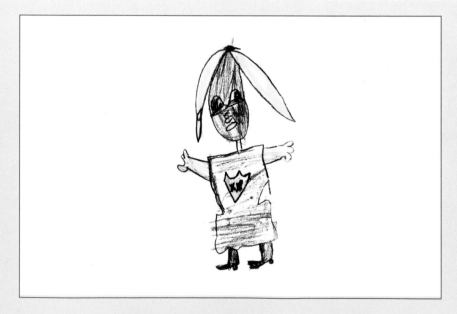

This picture is more expressive than his first one, with the arms opening to the world. However, a badge is still over the heart area.

The flower essences used during this phase included: **Agrimony, Clematis, Chestnut Bud, Mimulus, Holly, Cherry Plum, Rock Rose, Chicory, Crab Apple, Wild Oat, Heather, Cerato, Gentian, Larch, Hornbeam, Elm, Buttercup** and **Manzanita.**

Francisco Begins Art Lessons

After a break in the school year for several months, Francisco returned and was also able to begin art lessons. I was asked to formulate a new set of flower essences to help him prepare for the new school year.

Francisco reported that he was delighted with his art lessons and his teacher. Also, his home environment was calmer. His father had stopped drinking and his mother was also receiving therapy at Núcleo. I have noted that quite often, when one member of the family system begins to heal, the portal is opened for others to also grow and change.

Francisco expressed the wish to draw a portrait of me. Once again I could feel the projection of his soul in the drawing, and his feeling about my work with him through the flowers. This picture suggested his happiness as he continued to grow and be nourished by the life forces of nature. He drew me standing on the green earth with flowers on either side, embraced by trees and a shining sun, and a little rabbit. Elements of light and air are streaming though my hair.

The flowers used for Francisco during this time included **Walnut, Agrimony, Clematis, Chestnut Bud, Elm, Hornbeam, Gentian, Cerato, Heather, Mimulus, Crab Apple, Holly, Scleranthus, Wild Oat, Blackberry,** the **Learning Formula** (Rosemary, Shasta Daisy and Peppermint) and **Five-Flower Formula** (Star of Bethlehem, Impatiens, Clematis, Cherry Plum and Rock Rose). **Manzanita** was also used for him a few weeks later.

Following these sessions, Francisco showed remarkable stability and was able to discontinue all therapies at Núcleo Mãe Maria, including flower essence therapy. He now sees me only for "calibration" sessions, to maintain the good results he has achieved.

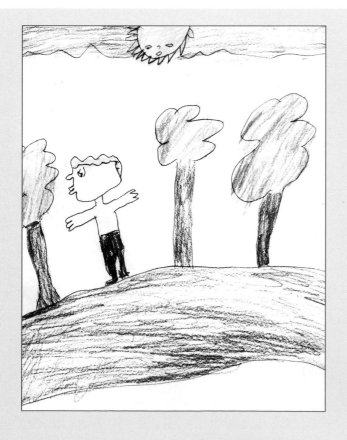

His soul is expressing a desire to receive and be connected with the forces of nature. He is standing on solid earth, surrounded by trees with the sun shining over him.

Felicidade — Francisco's Happiness as an Artist

Francisco flourished in his art work as well as other school work. By the end of the year, he had his first opportunity for a public show in Campinas. Francisco's art work captivated the public. His heart shines in a pure and simple way through his creative expressions, evoking beauty and innocence. Since his debut, Francisco has taken part in other exhibitions throughout the city. His artwork is so popular that it sells out immediately.

It is significant that Francisco has given the same name to all of his artwork: *Felicidade*. This name means happiness in Portuguese. Perhaps this single word is the greatest testament to the change in Francisco's soul.

It is truly amazing to consider the transformation in Francisco since the first time I met him. The layers of fear, low self-esteem and withdrawal from the world have melted away. Through his art, Francisco has found a way to shine in the world. His soul truly radiates happiness.

Francisco's art work captivated the public. His heart shines in a pure and simple way through his creative expressions, evoking beauty and innocence.

Felicidade means happiness in Portuguese. Perhaps this single word is the greatest testament to the change in Francisco's soul.

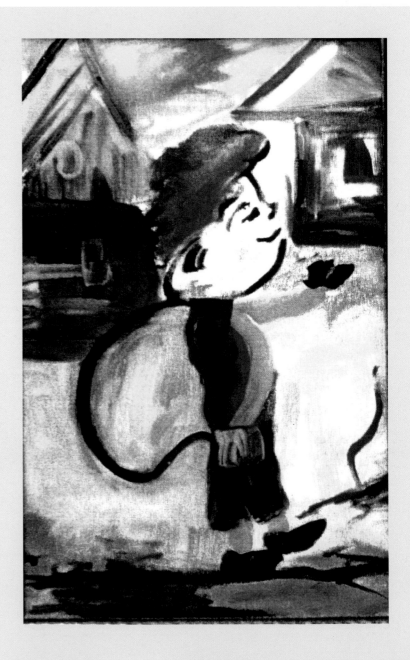

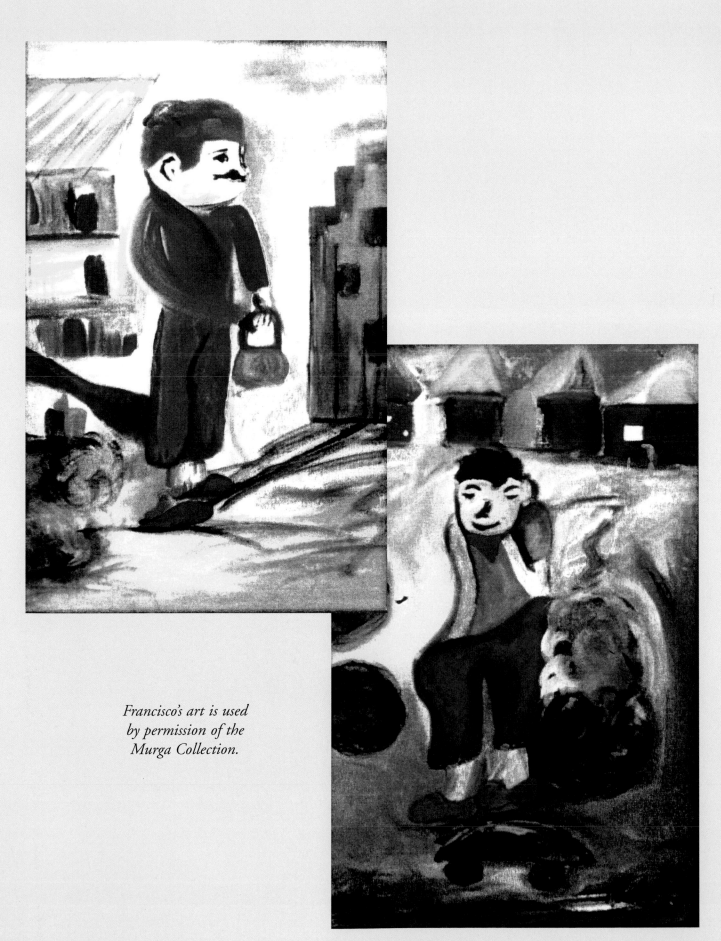

*Francisco's art is used
by permission of the
Murga Collection.*

Breaking New Ground:
Cuba is the First Nation to Incorporate Flower Essence Therapy in an Official Medical Program

by Beatriz M. Miyar, Ph.D.

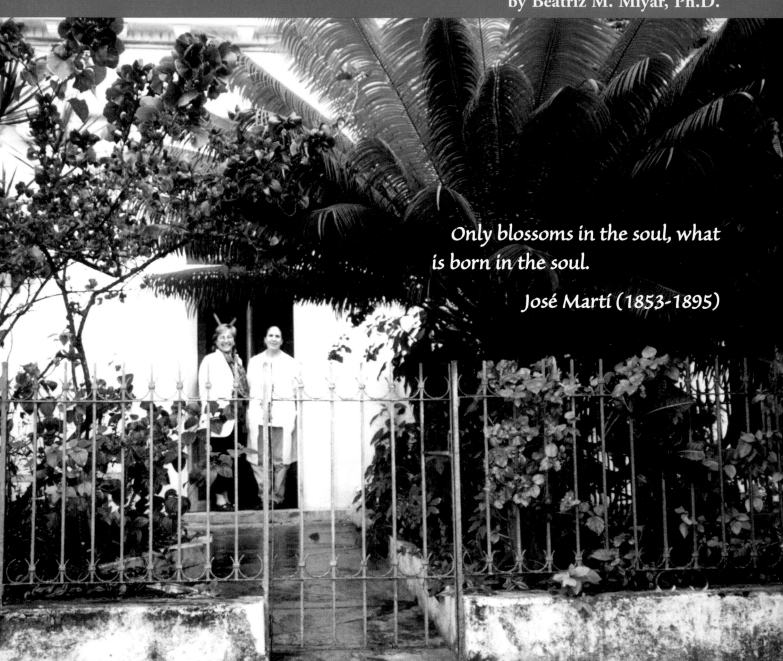

Only blossoms in the soul, what is born in the soul.

José Martí (1853-1895)

Dr. Sylvia Bustamante and Dr. Mirna Arrieta, at the entrance to the Natural and Traditional Medicine Clinic, affiliated with the Fajardo Hospital, Havana, Cuba

A major paradigm change within the medical profession is currently underway in Cuba, involving widespread application of holistic health modalities. Physicians and other health personnel, trained in Western conventional medicine, have gone beyond the limits of their previous education and practice. Flower Essence Therapy has gained recognition as one of the most important new healthcare programs in the Cuban medical establishment.

The following article is an edited summary of a report from Dr. Beatriz Miyar. It is based upon Dr. Miyar's dissertation, **Continuing Education in Cuban Healthcare: Holistic Medicine and Flower Essence Therapy** (Miyar, 2002).

The 1959 Revolution: Free and Accessible Healthcare

In 1959, Cuba had a relatively advanced medical infrastructure in comparison with other Latin American countries, however, the lower economic class and rural areas had little access to adequate healthcare. With only 6,000 doctors for a population of seven million, one medical school, and no national system for low-cost healthcare, the primary recipients of medical benefits were the affluent (Danielson, 1979). The 1959 Revolution brought needed social, political, and economic changes, including a massive restructuring of public healthcare through the creation of a unified comprehensive national healthcare system in the early 1960s. This system addressed the government's new policy of preventive medicine and free and accessible healthcare to all.

Campaigns to increase medical school enrollment, including compulsory rural and community service for newly graduated doctors, and community education in disease prevention and health awareness, flourished at that time. Dramatic results were evident in the last two decades of the 20th century, when Cuba attained a healthcare standard unprecedented in Latin America. This standard included modern healthcare facilities, the latest in biotechnology and a life expectancy of 76.0 years (MINSAP, 1999), compared to 76.7 in the United States (Centers for Disease Control and Prevention, 2001).

A thriving healthcare program was achieved through the Western scientific medical model, (Díaz-Briquets, 1983; Feinsilver, 1993). As long as hospital equipment and sufficient pharmaceutical drugs were available, combined with medical expertise, the practice of conventional medicine was successful. However, in 1989, the former Soviet Bloc disintegrated. Subsidies and financial resources to Cuba were terminated. The Cuban economy, including the healthcare system, suffered a devastating blow, with shortages in food, fuel, and supplies. Without sufficient funds, and in the face of a continued United States trade and economic embargo, the national healthcare system suffered a scarcity of medical supplies, technical equipment and pharmaceutical drugs. Faced with extremely adverse conditions for continued delivery of healthcare to a population now well accustomed to free and competent medical attention, the Cuban government made a resolute attempt to find new solutions.

The Resurgence of Natural and Traditional Medicine:

Defined as a "medical specialty" rather than "alternative"

Simultaneously, Cuba's long-standing involvement with natural and traditional medicine was experiencing a renaissance. Herbal medicine and hydro-mineral therapy had been practiced since early colonial times; homeopathy had been prevalent at the end of the 19th, and beginning of the 20th, centuries; and traditional Chinese medicine was introduced from Asia in the 1970s.

Cuban President Fidel Castro sought solutions for continued healthcare delivery. In 1991, he initiated a scientific research program to investigate commonly known Cuban medicinal plants (MINSAP, 1996). This announcement set off a chain of events that led to a policy pronouncement in 1995, *Directiva 26*. It officially established a general strategy for the development of natural and traditional medicine within the Ministry of Public Health and other agencies directly responsible for healthcare (MINSAP, 1996). This directive redefined the role of national health care by mandating the integration of holistic medicine within the established conventional system. The official interest in holistic medicine was not solely a result of economic duress – it also derived from a political commitment to support a healthy population.

The political goals remain to not only compensate for shortages of U.S. pharmaceutical drugs, but to develop a new Cuban model of natural holistic medicine which can be used in Cuba and in developing nations.

As they recognized the benefits of natural and traditional medicine, policy makers at the Cuban Ministry of Public Health began encouraging research. Healthcare professionals were steadily learning simple, yet remarkably effective and affordable, holistic medical therapies. They were reawakening traditional Cuban therapies and embracing other innovative health modalities introduced by visiting foreign professionals who supported Cuba in the face of the U.S. economic embargo and Soviet economic withdrawal.

In order to coordinate events and handle all programs necessary for the implementation and development of holistic medicine, as mandated by *Directiva 26*, a National Division of Natural and Traditional Medicine was established in 1995 under the Ministry of Public Health. Natural and traditional medicine was defined as a "medical specialty" rather than labeling it "alternative" (as holistic medicine is most frequently characterized in the United States). These specialties included

herbal medicine, homeopathy, traditional Chinese medicine, hydro-mineral therapy, hypnosis and relaxation exercises, therapeutic massage, physical therapy, ozone therapy, magnet therapy and other sources of natural energy (MINSAP, 1996).

Three years later, in January 1999, Flower Essence Therapy was added to this list. It is significant to note that in January 2002, a Resolution from the Executive Committee of the Council of Ministers mandated the further development of natural and traditional medicine. Resolution 4282 prioritized training as fundamental to the success of the program, and directed the Scientific Councils from Medical Schools to develop academic post-graduate studies, including Diplomate, Master and Doctorate degrees in Natural and Traditional Medicine (MINSAP, 2002).

According to Cuba's First Deputy Minister of Foreign Affairs, Fernando Remírez de Estenoz, the political goal was not merely to compensate for shortages of U.S. pharmaceutical drugs, but to develop a new model of natural holistic medicine for Cuba and for other developing nations. These innovative strategies would allow Cuba to achieve improved health and self-sufficiency and become less dependent on the world market (2001).

History of Flower Essence Therapy in Cuba

During the years of 1992-1994, Eduardo Grecco and Barbara Espeche, Argentinean authors and psychologists, held conferences for 200 Cuban physicians at a medical school institute in Havana and donated books and flower essences. Similar actions were taken by Maria Dolores Paoli de Souza, a Venezuelan psychologist and energy medicine therapist, and Antonio Duek, a Mexican architect.

Pioneering Cuban physicians began treating patients and incorporating Flower Essence Therapy into their practices, observing positive results with their patients. This period reflects a special time in the history of Cuban society when, along with the termination of the Soviet Bloc subsidies, Cuban professionals searched eagerly for innovative ideas to meet the resulting challenges. They were trained to be proactive in conducting scientific research in order to directly verify their clinical observations. This professional demeanor contributed greatly to the development of the Flower Essence Therapy movement.

There are approximately 64,000 doctors in Cuba, and few had any previous formal training in holistic medicine, including Flower Essence Therapy. In 1997, Dr. Concepción Campa Huergo, Director of *Instituto Finlay*, and one of Cuba's most prominent researchers, collaborated with the Ministry of Public Health to invite two Argentinean professors to teach the first official course in Flower Essence Therapy. By October 1998, there were 104 graduates, with 25 research studies showing notable results in treating various physical and psychological pathologies such as migraines, depression, skin conditions, menopause, stress and asthma.

Faced with such encouraging results and better trained Flower Essence practitioners, the Ministry of Public Health authorities officially recognized Flower Essence Therapy in January 1999, as a valid medical modality to be integrated into the national health system. This recognition took Flower Essence Therapy to another level by freeing all health professionals to apply it in their practices.

> The Ministry of Public Health authorities officially recognized Flower Essence Therapy as a valid medical modality to be integrated into the national health system.

Voices of the Practitioners

"First, we experiment with ourselves, and then we take this healing experience to others. I consider this a new paradigm because I learned from personal experience."

During my time spent in Cuba documenting the First National Flower Essence Program in 2000, I informally interviewed numerous practitioners in a qualitative research approach. The final selection of 23 professionals for the "interview group" was guided by three criteria:

1) key informants who knew enough about the phenomenon of Flower Essence Therapy to identify its most motivating aspects,
2) thoughtful practitioners able to share their personal histories and experiences with the therapy,
3) a sample representative of the medical personnel involved with Flower Essence Therapy, including the variables of gender, age, racial origin, and branch of professional training.

The motivation expressed by the interview group may be divided into three categories:

1) *professional motivation* — dissatisfaction with inadequacies of Western medicine, ability to better treat emotional dimensions of afflictions, better quality of healthcare, no side-effects, gentle;
2) *personal motivation* — individual experience of illness and cure and affinity for natural medicines;
3) *practical motivation* — cost-effectiveness, patient demand, good results with Flower Essence Therapy.

Most of the Cuban professionals had arrived at crossroads in their careers: Western medical schooling was not showing the results they were taught to expect. In seeking solutions, Dr. Pablo, an internal medicine physician, noted, "I felt a kinship with the influences of change that had been taking place in the West during the last twenty years. This created an interest in holistic treatments…inspired by the new physics, transpersonal psychology, biology, as well as other informational sciences."

Concerning the frequent negative side effects of Western pharmaceutical drugs, Dr. Lela, a specialist doctor in health administration, said, "Flower Essence Therapy is more natural and health-enhancing, and it frees the patient from taking intoxicating chemical drugs."

Dr. Felicidad, a long-established psychiatrist, commented, "I suffered from a respiratory allergy for seven years, which was cured with Flower Essence Therapy. First, we experiment with ourselves, and then we take this healing experience to others. I consider this a new paradigm because I learned from personal experience. Based on this, I learned how to become a better therapist and to understand patient response."

Patient Demand Spurs a "Bottom Up" Movement

Although the majority of the interview group was unanimous in experiencing a personal change in their approach to healthcare, most of them were hesitant to say the movement had brought a paradigm shift within the Cuban national health system. Dr. Felicidad stated, "It is not yet a movement big enough to change the whole paradigm of the health institutions and their administrators, but this does not renounce the existence of more open-minded persons." Looking at trends in the institutionalization of Flower Essence Therapy, nineteen from the interview group saw the Flower Essence Therapy movement as a profound and irreversible paradigm shift within their individual professional practice and gave the following reasons:
☆ encourages a better approach in the health professional,
☆ offers a more humanistic approach to medicine
☆ receives official support,
☆ complements Western medicine,
☆ is scientifically validated,
☆ helps the patient,
☆ is more cost-efficient.

Four interviewees did not consider Flower Essence Therapy a paradigm shift, giving these reasons: it is a slow change, many do not believe in it, and it is not a sufficiently large movement. They added that conducting more scientific research in this field was necessary to establish a fundamental change.

Multiple research studies involving Cuban medical professionals are regularly taking place with noteworthy results. One of these studies, conducted in a Havana hospital, demonstrated the positive effects of Flower Essence Therapy with severely affected psychiatric patients. Four hundred schizophrenics and neurotics were treated with flower essences from August 1996 through June 1999 (Bustamante, 2001). (*See practitioner profiles and case studies at the end of this article.*)

Regarding trends for the dissemination of Flower Essence Therapy amongst Cuban health professionals, the entire interview group agreed that *patient demand* was a crucial factor spurring this "bottom-up" movement. Another strong consensus involved commitment to better quality of healthcare, with a gradual expansion in interest amongst a majority of medical professionals. Although many prefer to continue using the more established conventional methods, these physicians are increasingly referring patients they are not able to help — for example, cases involving asthma and high blood pressure) — to Natural and Traditional Medicine Clinics for treatment with Flower Essence Therapy.

Going Beyond a Biochemical Model of Healing

Reaction to anything new and unknown can be expected. Some professionals sought to understand the scientific validity of the new practice and were concerned about quality control. This type of resistance, as explained by a Cuban physicist, is usually an inability to, "go beyond observing the human body as solely a biochemical, mechanistic Newtonian model where Science is … a compilation of statistics and experiments drawn from an inorganic world." Political and cultural resistance also occurred for those unwilling to change for various reasons — fear, jealousy, disbelief, skepticism, and defense of privilege or "turf."

Dr. Pablo commented, "To practice this new approach to medicine, one needs flexibility and courage. This means that we have to shed many aspects of our current belief system ... it implies a nearly 180-degree change from the concepts and convictions that previously sustained us. Not many therapists and doctors have been capable of carrying things to this extreme, yet I still consider that a wholehearted embrace of this new paradigm is the only possible solution."

Arcoiris de Cuba: Cuba's Floral Rainbow

In the spring of 1999, Dr. Julia Nancy Martínez Fundora, an established flower essence practitioner, announced her three-year research results on the development of native Cuban essences. After being guided by a spiritual feeling to go into nature and observe plants, she embarked upon the study of Botanical Sciences. Dr. Martínez credits the Creator and Nature for her ability to identify the forty-five flower essences from Cuba that compose the Arcoiris de Cuba (Cuba's Rainbow).

During her presentation at the Cuban Congress on Flower Essence Therapy in October 1999, Dr. Martínez attributed her inspiration to Dr. Bach and Cuba's abundant and beautiful array of wildflowers. *Arcoiris de Cuba* essences are currently undergoing a scientific validation process.

In the Fields of Practice: "Doctor, I Feel So Good"

As part of my doctoral research, I frequently visited two Natural and Traditional Medical Clinics affiliated with hospitals in Havana. Each have an exclusive area for Flower Essence Therapy consultation. I observed the daily practice of Flower Essence Therapy and met patients who reported their positive experiences, along with flower essence practitioners. When asked to comment on how they felt, patients were eager to express themselves. Sample comments include:

This therapy has changed my life by helping me transform my outlook. I was able to eliminate most stress and feel peace within.

I have found an answer to a health condition I had for years that other doctors were unable to help me with.

These flowers have helped me where I could not get relief before.

I have been treated with Flower Essence Therapy for some time. Not only my original condition has improved, but other aspects of my life have gotten better, too.

Similar comments from clinics throughout Cuba indicate that Flower Essence Therapy is a grass roots movement. I observed therapist-patient relationships to be intimate, humane, spiritual, and caring, while remaining professional and objective. Doctors are extremely committed and hardworking in a health system where all services are provided at no cost to the patient. I witnessed patients bearing gifts of appreciation to their

From Dr. Pérez's study described on page 88: "The study found that except for the bipolar dysfunctions, the rest of the psychiatric pathologies improved with the administration of floral therapy. The consumption of pharmaceutical medications was greatly diminished. All of the patients improved their quality of life after six months of therapy."

> *I saw the therapist-patient relationship as intimate, humane, spiritual, and caring, while remaining professional and objective. Doctors are extremely committed and hardworking, in a health system where all services are provided at no cost to the patient.*

practitioners, such as homemade desserts, freshly brewed Cuban coffee, honey, mangoes, oranges, fresh flowers, plants, books, writing notebooks, pens, and brandy for preparing flower essence dosage bottles.

Cuban hospitals receive their budgets, which include supplies and salaries, from the Ministry of Public Health. Patients obtain essences at pharmacies by presenting a prescription from a doctor or a psychologist, or directly from a practitioner at participating clinics. Remedies are prepared from matrix sets acquired from different areas of the world, and from the national set, Arcoiris de Cuba.

Training and Establishment of Flower Essence Therapy

Continuing professional education has helped to consolidate the knowledge base necessary for changing perspectives in medical practice. Self-directed learning has also nurtured the movement. A variety of workshops have been conducted to train practitioners and to provide a critical forum for exchange of information.

In Cuba, education is cost-free to students, there is no private medical practice and all medical personnel are state-employed. Continuing professional education can be roughly divided into two areas: first, academic programs earning Doctorate, Master, or Specialist degrees; and second, "non-academic" studies such as diplomate courses, and training. Both types require a full eight years of general medical education or a four-year Bachelor's degree and are supervised by the Ministry of Public Health and the Ministry of Higher Education. The diplomate is the apex of the non-

academic side of continuing professional education. Diplomate programs enjoy wide enrollment from medical professionals who must attend a minimum of 250 hours of study and clinical practice in order to receive a recognized Diplomate certificate status.

State officials and administrators have the power to accredit any particular body of knowledge within Cuba's twenty-one medical schools. At the time of my dissertation, there were ten officially recognized Diplomate programs in the area of natural and traditional medicine for doctors, dentists and nurses, including homeopathy, behavioral medicine, physical therapy and rehabilitation, acupuncture and herbal medicine. Since Flower Essence Therapy was officially sanctioned in 1999, advocates have worked to have it recognized as a separate medical specialty worthy of Diplomate certificate status. In the first National Flower Essence Program 2000, 1450 medical professionals throughout Cuba, received a six-month training equivalent to that required for Diplomate certification.

The strategy for institutionalization of Flower Essence Therapy training consists of progressing through the levels of the medical education structure in Cuba (see figure below), starting from a base of self-directed learning and practitioner initiative. The movement is now situated between levels III and IV. At least one entity — *Instituto Finlay* — has experimented with a Diplomate sequence, although a permanent Diplomate has not been established and there are no graduate courses leading to higher degrees in Flower Essence Therapy within the medical school.

Looking Toward the Future: Recommendations for Practice

The following recommendations for practice are based on the findings of the study and can ensure more successful development of holistic medicine:

☆ continue to carefully manage, evaluate and document the processes and results of Flower Essence Therapy training,

☆ appoint experienced and knowledgeable medical personnel in Flower Essence Therapy and holistic medicine to decision-making administrative positions,

☆ develop a comprehensive curriculum in Flower Essence Therapy at the level of academic and medical schools,

☆ allocate more budgetary resources for Flower Essence Therapy,

☆ ensure that Flower Essence Therapy is available to the entire population.

Concluding Remarks: A Tribute to Cuba's Flower Essence Therapy Practitioners

The Cuban practitioners who are pioneers in the field of Flower Essence Therapy are motivated by factors beyond their medical training, politics, and social conditioning. They embrace a holistic philosophy that reaches outside their professional practice, permeating every aspect of life. The success of these pioneers is due to more than exterior qualifications. These practitioners reflected on what they could do to improve the art of healing, and they were transformed in the process. This process gave birth to a bottom-up movement, which eventually secured official governmental recognition of Flower Essence Therapy within the national health system. They were guided by the fundamental values within Cuba's unique national healthcare system, where health services are a birthright offered free of charge; and innovation in healthcare is encouraged.

These medical pioneers have developed a wider vision for healing, and a more encompassing understanding of human identity. They have become deeply involved with their patients, resulting in a more caring patient-doctor relationship. One especially sees in Flower Essence Therapy, that medical professionals work *with* the patient, but not *for* the patient, providing the tools for patients to heal themselves.

Copyright © Beatriz M. Miyar, Ph.D.

Pyramid strategy of institutionalization of Flower Essence Therapy and associated professional education realms not yet reached (indicated by dotted lines).

Bibliography

Bustamante Rodríguez, S., MD (2001, September). *Una mirada al futuro: el desarrollo de medicina natural y tradicional en Cuba*. Paper presented at the 2001 Meeting of the Latin American Studies Association, Washington, D.C.

Centers for Disease Control and Prevention (CDC). (2001). *National Center for Health Statistics*. Maryland: U.S. Department of Health and Human Services.

Danielson, R. (1979). *Cuban medicine*. New Brunswick, NJ: Transaction.

Books

Díaz-Briquets, S. (1983). *Health revolution in Cuba*. Austin: University of Texas Press.

Martí, J. (1975). Cuadernos de apuntes. *Obras Completas* (2nd ed.), *21*(3). Cuba: Editorial Ciencias Sociales.

Ministerio de Salud Pública (MINSAP) (Ministry of Public Health). (1996). *Programa nacional para el desarrollo y generalización de la medicina natural y tradicional* (National program for the development of natural and traditional medicine). La Habana, Cuba: MINSAP.

Ministerio de Salud Pública (MINSAP) (Ministry of Public Health). (1999). *Annual health statistics report 1999*. La Habana, Cuba: Ministry of Public Health, National Health Statistics Bureau, UNICEF.

Ministerio de Salud Pública (MINSAP) (Ministry of Public Health). (1999). *Health care situation in Cuba – basic indicators 1999*. La Habana, Cuba: Ministry of Public Health, World Health Organization, Pan American Health Organization.

Ministerio de Salud Pública (MINSAP) (Ministry of Public Health). (2002).
Resolution No. 4282 Medicina Natural Tradicional. La Habana, Cuba: MINSAP.

Miyar, Beatriz M., Ph.D. (2002). *Continuing Education in Cuban Healthcare: Holistic Medicine and Flower Essence Therapy*. Doctoral dissertation. Florida State University.

Remírez de Estenoz, F., MD (2001, April). *The Cuban health care system*. Paper presented at the Broad International Lecture Series. Florida State University, Tallahassee, Florida.

For a copy of Dr. Miyar's full dissertation or more information about her work contact her at bmm15@earthlink.net

About Dr. Beatriz Miyar

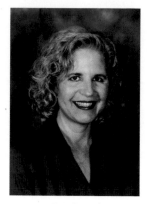

Beatriz M. Miyar, Ph.D. was born in Cuba. She was introduced to natural and traditional medicine when she was only 40 days old and the family doctor successfully treated her for colic with herbal infusions.

She received a B.A. degree in International Affairs and an M.S. degree in International Intercultural Development Education from Florida State University, and has worked as a human resource director, gemologist, teacher, healer, event producer and college instructor. She has traveled extensively worldwide and has done fieldwork in Cuba, Mexico and Peru. Dr. Miyar describes her multi-faceted life as being dedicated to experiencing the love and peace that lie within each of us and to helping others in a holistic manner.

In autumn 2002, Dr. Miyar was awarded her Ph.D. in Education at Florida State University in Tallahassee, Florida, based on her dissertation research project: ***Continuing Education in Cuban Healthcare: Holistic Medicine and Flower Essence Therapy***. Her doctoral dissertation allowed her to combine her research interests in the areas of international education policy, continuing education in alternative and holistic medicine, and healthcare policy. Dr. Miyar traveled to her homeland to conduct interviews, document the training sessions of the Program, visit medical practices at a variety of institutions, and attend the VII International Congress of Flower Essence Therapists held in La Habana. She was warmly welcomed as a researcher and friend by Ministry of Public Health officials, medical professionals, and patients.

Dr. Miyar returns periodically to Cuba to do further research. Officials and practitioners continue to express amazement that professional interest in flower essence training is growing faster than they had expected or could have imagined.

Profiles of Cuban Flower Essence Therapists

Dr. Pedro Sastriques and Dr. Xonia Lopez

Dr. Pedro Sastriques Silva and his wife Dr. Xonia López Cepero are two of the leading flower essence practitioners in Cuba. Dr. Sastriques is a medical internist and Dr. Lopez is a pediatrician. Both of them utilize holistic medicine, including flower essence therapy, in their busy practices in Cuba's capital city, Havana. They are affiliated with the Bioenergetic and Flower Essence Therapy Department at the Psychiatric Hospital of Havana, and the International Oncology Clinic, National Institute of Oncology, also in Havana. Dr. Sastriques has also studied Anthroposophic Medicine, through the assistance of Dr. Michaela Glockler, Director of the Anthroposophic Medical Section at the Goetheanum, Dornach, Switzerland.

Since 1996, Sastriques and Lopez have developed a system of energetic testing through kinesiology, known as EEI – Evaluación Enérgetica Integrativa (Integrative Energetic Evaluation). EEI is a kinesiological approach using the Arm Reflex as a neuromuscular reflex. Dr. Sastriques describes it as a method for obtaining "information from both cerebral hemispheres," guiding the patient to identify important past events that have condi-

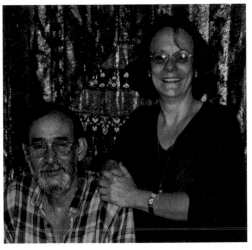

Dr. Pedro Sastriques and Dr. Xonia Lopez

tioned and reinforced present emotional states. They also integrate the insights and methods of Wilhelm Reich and Carl Jung in their therapy.

Drs. Sastriques and Lopez conduct research with students at la Escuela Nacional de Arte (National School of Art) where all students receive flower essences during their four-year course of study, to address emotional blocks that interfere with the creative process.

In their outpatient clinic at the Psychiatric Hospital of Havana, four doctors treat approximately 60 patients daily with bioenergetic testing, flower essences and botanical medicine. From their office in the National Institute of Oncology, they use flower essences to alleviate despair, pain and suffering among patients in the final stages of illness.

Flower essences are a "liquid conscience" for awareness and transcendence of life's problems. ... They enable the patient to take an active role when faced with personality problems. In this manner, flower essence therapy assists with any healing process.

Dr. Pedro Sastriques

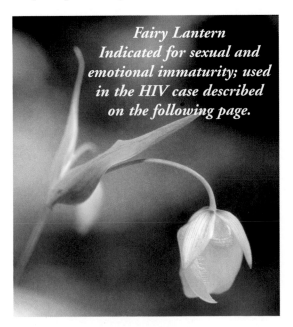

*Fairy Lantern
Indicated for sexual and emotional immaturity; used in the HIV case described on the following page.*

A case from Dr. Pedro Sastriques

HIV-positive man deals with fear and depression

A 31-year old male, who worked in the tourism industry, saw Dr. Sastriques at the outpatient clinic in the Department of Bioenergetics and Flower Essence Therapy.

The initial visit indicated a number of physical ailments, including a hiatal hernia, and the patient was emotionally distraught, bordering on depression. Afraid of intimacy, he did not express his true feelings for fear of not being understood. He had an erratic, disorganized life. His first combination was **Pink Monkeyflower**, **Self-Heal**, **Morning Glory**, **Red Clover** and **Heather**, selected by the EEI method, and taken orally in combination. (These selection and administration methods were used for all subsequent formulas.)

By the time of his next visit, one month later, his condition had worsened with a diagnosis of HIV-positive (asymptomatic). Now he was dealing with panic and nervous collapse. He started to face his erratic and immature sexual and emotional behavior, his possessiveness of his partner, and self-destructiveness. His new formula was **Red Clover**, **Scarlet Monkeyflower**, **Lady's Slipper**, **Fairy Lantern**, **Black Cohosh**, **Mustard** and **Pink Monkeyflower**.

Therapy continued for three-and-a-half years, with a total of eight sessions. The patient encountered depression, sexual repression and guilt, shame, alienation, fatigue, and disorientation, as well as digestive problems and insomnia. By the end of the second year of therapy, he began facing deep emotional pain from childhood traumas, working through resistance, hostility and numbness of feeling, in order to be able to forgive the past.

Mid-way into his third year of therapy, he began feeling more secure and able to progressively encounter social situations. He was no longer depressed, though he had periods of fear and vulnerability. As his therapy progressed, he dealt with tension between his sexuality and a developing spirituality, hypersensitivity, and low self-esteem.

Flower essences in that combination were **Pink Yarrow**, **Easter Lily**, **Buttercup**, **Oak** and **Angelica**.

Flower essence therapy is continuing, with no other medical treatments and no pharmaceutical drugs. The patient attends lectures and group therapy sessions, and has regular serological checkups at a conventional medical clinic. His condition is stable, and the improvement has been confirmed by the observations of his family and friends.

A case from Dr. Xonia López

A physician comes to terms with fatherhood

A 39-year old male physician came to the clinic complaining of stress and anguish, lack of concentration, insomnia, feeling burdened, and nervousness. During his first session, it became clear that a key element underlying his emotional tension and low self-esteem was a conflict with authority stemming from an erratic relationship with his father. He was given **Chamomile**, **Saguaro**, **Pretty Face**, **Cerato** and **Corn**, selected by the EEI method.

Over the next half-year, he had a total of five sessions, in which he worked progressively through his repressed childhood and adolescent emotions. He began to realize that the recent birth of his own son had triggered painful memories of his own alcoholic father, which made it difficult to take responsibility for his own family.

By the fifth session, he was experiencing solid change, wanting to eliminate false images and identities that did not serve him, and to free himself of past influences. He was dealing with his resistance to change, hypersensitivity, and a tendency toward indulgence and obesity as a protection for his vulnerability, using a formula of **Sagebrush**, **Pomegranate**, **Olive** and **Yarrow**.

No pharmaceutical drugs nor other treatments were given. The patient, as well as his family and friends, noted his improvement, although he was previously unfamiliar with flower essence therapy.

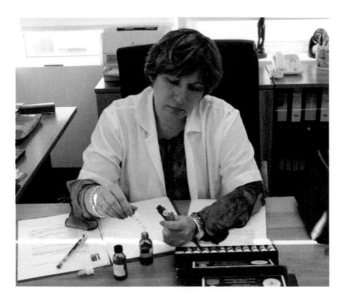

Psychologist Haydée Ramos

Elvira Haydée Ramos González is a psychologist at the Psychiatry Department of the Hospital and Medical Institute "Calixto García." She has participated in national and international events as a participant and presenter and is an active participant in the FES Depression Study, providing over a hundred cases using the Beck and Hamilton scales.

A case from Haydée Ramos

Recovering from childhood asthma and rape

A 45-year old female patient suffered asthma since she was 8 years old. She received psychiatric treatment three times and was sexually violated at 17. She reported feeling very irritable, arguing with her alcoholic husband and two daughters. She was diagnosed with liver cirrhosis, had gastritis and experienced frequent chest pain. She was on medication for her asthma.

Over a period of six-and-a-half months, she was given the following flower essences, in various combinations, as her condition evolved: **Willow, Beech, Dandelion, Yerba Santa, Manzanita, Self-Heal, Crab Apple, Impatiens, Star of Bethlehem, Holly** and **Pine**. Besides her physical ailments, she dealt with feelings of ugliness and impurity. She underwent regression therapy, in which she dealt with the sexual violation and the childhood onset of her asthma.

As a result of her therapy, most of her original symptoms were alleviated, except for her gastritis. Asthma attacks became infrequent and she stopped taking all pharmaceutical drugs, except for an asthma spray. Her liver cirrhosis cleared by the end of the therapy, with a normal reading for her ALT (Alanine Transaminase) test.

Her relationship with her husband and daughters improved, and they noticed that she was more calm and less irritable.

My personal philosophy is that Flower Essence Therapy helps to understand the symptoms or sickness, thus helping to heal the soul.

Lic. Haydée Ramos

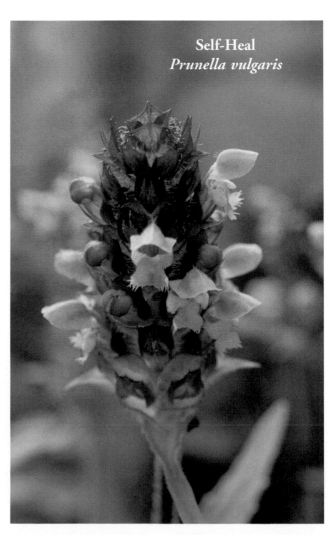

Self-Heal
Prunella vulgaris

Dr. Silvia Bustamante

Dr. Silvia Bustamante is a medical doctor (University of Havana, 1970) and specialist in psychiatry (Cuban Ministry of Public Health, 1976). She has conducted research with the Cuban Academy of Sciences, with extensive post-graduate study in psychiatry, hypnosis, acupuncture, flower essence therapy, anthroposophic medicine and Reiki.

Dr. Bustamante turned to natural and traditional medicine—especially Flower Essence Therapy—in 1996, after she personally experienced its benefits. Presently, she is the director of the Natural and Traditional Medicine Clinic of the Hospital Comandante Manuel Fajardo in Havana, Cuba, where she continues to see patients and teach holistic medicine courses to health professionals. She uses the EEI (Integrated Energetic Evaluation) system of Drs. Sastriques and Lopez for diagnosis and flower essence selection.

"I consider Flower Essence Therapy a holistic method that allows us to view human beings in all their dimensions and to treat the physical, emotional, mental and spiritual aspects. It is the only method that allows us to use the dictates of the soul for learning during this incarnation."

Dr. Silvia Bustamante

A Case from Dr. Silvia Bustamante

A woman recovers from depression after the death of a colleague

A woman, who had suffered chronic depression throughout her life, became extremely distraught due to the death of a work colleague. As her condition worsened, she began taking the pharmaceutical drugs she had previously used, but this time she did not get better. This was the reason she came to the Flower Essence Therapy clinic.

During the clinical interview she expressed much fear of being alone at home, nostalgia and great sadness. She felt unloved and unappreciated, and frequently recalled the death of a beloved work colleague. **Mimulus** was chosen for fear, **Honeysuckle** for nostalgia, **Mustard** for deep sadness, **Arnica** for past traumas, and **Evening Primrose** for feeling unloved, accompanied by general depression and trauma. The essences were taken for a period of six months, combined with relaxation and breathing exercises.

The patient showed noticeable improvement, and after a month, was able to return to work. (She had been away from her job for 6 months.) All symptoms of fear and depression disappeared two months later, as confirmed by the observations of her relatives and work colleagues.

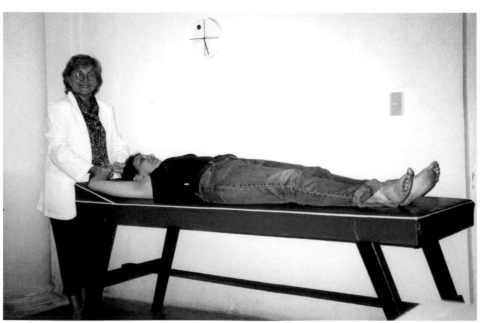

Dr. Bustamante testing a patient with the EEI system

Dr. Maribel Pérez

Dr. Maribel Pérez López is a Specialist in Psychiatry and Social Psychiatry and Director of the Clinic for Psychosomatic Imbalances, Stress, and Sexual Dysfunction at the Hospital and Medical Institute "Joaquín Albarrán Domínguez," Havana, Cuba. She has presented many graduate-level courses on flower essence therapy, alcoholism, hypnosis and hypnotic regression at Cuban hospitals. She frequently presents scientific papers at professional conferences on psychiatry, hypnosis, alcoholism and flower essence therapy, and has published papers in numerous medical journals.

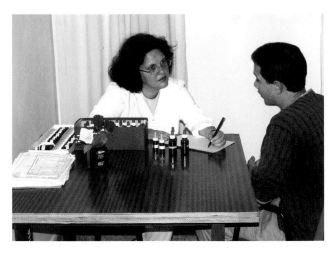

"At first, I believed that Flower Essence Therapy would not work, but immediately thereafter, I began seeing its benefits for my patients' health. ... Today, both psychiatrists and other doctors frequently refer cases to me." — *Dr. Maribel Pérez*

A Case from Dr. Maribel Pérez
Overcoming resentment and blame

A 35-year old single woman was a licensed medical technician, although she worked as a receptionist at the Ministry of Agriculture. Her initial symptoms included restlessness, aggressiveness, and difficulty in concentrating. She felt resentful that she had not been able to practice her career, and blamed her aunt for all her misfortunes. She often expressed her hatred for her mother and aunt by physically hitting them, and had conflicts with others, including her psychiatrists. Her father died of a heart attack when she was 15 and also, during her adolescence, she was diagnosed with psychosis.

Her flower essence therapy spanned two and a half years, with six different flower essence combinations. She started with **Hornbeam**, **Mimulus**, **Impatiens**, **Holly** and **Star of Bethlehem** for fear, hatred, impatience, and losses in life such as father, friends, career, and mental health, along with mental exhaustion.

Midway in her therapy, she used a combination of **Holly**, **Willow**, **Chestnut Bud**, **Cherry Plum** and **Clematis** for a period of 20 months. During this time, her resentment and hatred towards her aunt became more evident and she had conflicts at work with her boss. Clematis and Cherry Plum helped to orient her to the present and addressed her impulsiveness and lack of self-control. Chestnut Bud was used to help her reflect upon and to learn from her experience. During this time she asked her aunt for forgiveness, her work relations improved, and she began working and studying for another career. She began to regret the time she has lost in her life due to her condition.

Her improvement continued as she became determined to live, find a partner, and approach daily living with a fuller acceptance of her real possibilities. Her last formula of **Lotus**, **Golden Ear Drops**, **Sunflower** and **Mariposa Lily** was used to bring harmony and self-realization. She wanted to increase her spiritual consciousness and continue to transform her many difficulties and traumas

As a result of her therapy, she was able to discontinue the drug carbamazepine, which she had been taking at a dosage of 200 mg per day. She was able to eliminate resentment and hatred, and become more responsive to life challenges. She realized and analyzed her mistakes, and now leads a normal life as an adult. Her mother, aunt, and work colleagues have all acknowledged these changes.

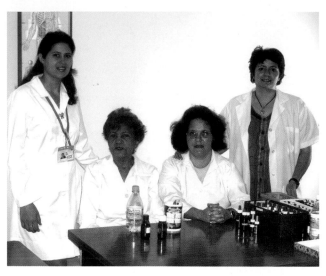

Dr. Maribel Pérez (second from the right) with colleagues at the Hospital and Medical Institute "Joaquín Albarrán Domínguez"

A Scientific Study by Dr. Maribel Pérez

A year-long clinical study

● From January to December in 2000, 207 participant cases were studied via consultations at the J. Albarrán hospital's psychiatric consultation service.

● Each patient was analyzed according to clinical history, personal history, psychological tests: Cattel (Anxiety) and Zung (Depression), a "Quality of Life" survey and family interviews.

● The following clinical, psychological and social variables were considered: a) Age, b) Sex, c) Race, d) Occupation, e) Educational Level, f) Marital Status, g) Personal Pathological Records, h) Depression, i) Anxiety, and j) Social Relations.

Married women in their middle years

● Patients were in the age range of 31 to 60 years, in which people generally show an increase in responsibilities, very active daily jobs, social and family lives, and more vulnerability to suffering from a variety of psychiatric illnesses.

● A prevalence of women existed in the sample. Men are culturally conditioned to avoid consultation with psychologists and psychiatrists; they only seek help in the event of extreme necessity.

● The larger part of the population has a mid to high range of schooling, which corresponds with the general population possessing a high level of education.

● Married persons were predominant in the sample for both sexes, constituting 60.3% of the sample.

● Race was not significant with regard to the population's distribution, nor in the results of the study.

Decreased use of pharmaceuticals and excellent results with flower essences

● The 32 cases treated for Major Depression initially took one dose of 50 mg of a tricyclic antidepressant. During the three months of treatment with flower essence therapy, they continued with the same dose, although the symptomological picture had already improved. Within six months, 65% of the patients received only flower remedies since their depressive symptoms had disappeared.

● Customary doses of antidepressants were given, but the typical worsening of the clinical pictures did not occur after six months. These patients continued flower essence therapy treatment for two more years to lessen the possibility of relapse.

● Those patients with bipolar dysfunctions achieved a slight improvement during six months of combined treatment. We surmise that this condition requires more treatment time with flower essence therapy.

● All of those with neurotic dysfunctions eliminated the need for psycho-pharmaceutical intervention very rapidly. Within three months of therapy, they had the ability to make deep changes within their personality with significant insight into their personal histories.

● Patients with situational dysfunctions progressed similarly.

● Clients suffering from schizophrenia had a customary dose of antipsychotic (neuroleptic) drugs, along with flower essence therapy. At the end of three months, 60% were involved in their social lives. Three months later, 100% had been able to decrease the doses of anti-psychotic drugs, and maintained quality social and family lives.

● Personality dysfunctions behaved similarly to situational and neurotic dysfunctions. Within three months, they showed signs of improvement in behavioral patterns.

● For psychosomatic dysfunctions, there was a 90% success rate. These patients controlled their pathology through flower essence therapy only.

● Patients suffering from dysfunctions caused by alcoholism used flower essence therapy almost entirely, without relapses, for six months.

A cost-benefit analysis was included in the study that compared the relative costs of flower essence therapy compared to treatment with conventional anti-depressants and tranquilizers. Dr. Perez found that flower essence therapy was much less expensive.

The full study (in the original Spanish or in English translation) is available from the Flower Essence Society: *Influencia Terapéutica de las Esencias Florales en los Pacientes con Enfermedades Clasificadas Como Psiquiátricas y Psicosomáticas*, Servicio de Psiquiatría "René Yodú Prevez" Hospital Docente Investigativo Clínico Quirúrgico Joaquín Albarrán, Havana, Cuba, 2001. *(Therapeutic Influence of Flower Essences in Patients with Illnesses Classified as Psychiatric and Psychosomatic.)*

Five Clinical Studies Demonstrate the Effectiveness of Flower Essence Therapy in the Treatment of Depression

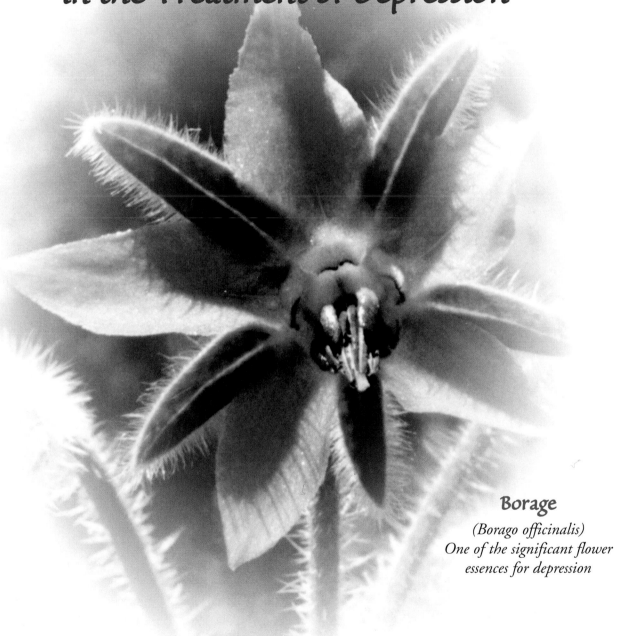

Borage
(Borago officinalis)
One of the significant flower essences for depression

In the midst of winter, I finally learned that there was in me an invincible summer. — Albert Camus, *Actuelles*

A Convergence of Evidence:

Flower Essence Therapy in the Treatment of Major Depression

an analysis by Dr. Jeffrey R. Cram,

with data from Dr. Pedro Sastriques Silva, Lic. Elvira Haydée Ramos González,
Dr. María de los Ángeles Fernández de la Llera, and Dr. Sol Inés Tena Rodríguez

The convergence of findings from these five outcome studies strongly supports the concept that flower essences may be used adjunctively to facilitate the resolution of mild to moderate depression.

Abstract

This article presents the findings of a series of studies conducted to determine the clinical efficacy of flower essences on the treatment of mild to moderate depression. Funding for the study was provided by the Flower Essence Society. Therapists participating in the study did so on a volunteer basis.

Five independent clinical outcome studies are presented, each lending evidence towards understanding the clinical effects of flower essences on the treatment of depression. The results of these studies were measured using the Beck Depression Inventory (BDI) and the Hamilton Depression Scale (HAM-D). A time series analysis of the data was conducted using an ANOVA (analysis of variance) for repeated measures. Four of the studies were conducted by therapists in Cuba under the auspices of the Cuban Ministry of Public Health. The first of these studies examined over 100 patients, of which approximately half completed therapy. They were tracked over a period of five months, with an outcome indicating a significant reduction in depressive symptoms. The second and third studies utilized 20 patient/subjects and examined the effects of flower essence therapy over a 2-month and 3-month period of time. Again, significant drops in depression scores were noted during the first month, with further decreases during the second and third months. Both studies show reductions of the BDI total score of 76-77%. The fourth study utilized 24 cases over a 3-month period of time. Significant decreases in depressions were noted for the first two months, with this stabilizing at a 60 to 80% reduction during the third month.

The fifth study entailed a multi-site clinical trial conducted in the United States. It has been published elsewhere (Cram, 2001b). This study of 12 depressed subjects included a one-month baseline followed by 3 months of treatment that entailed usual care along with flower essence therapy. The findings indicated a stable baseline, followed by a 50% reduction in depression scores when flower essence therapy was introduced. This clinical change was maintained over a period of 3 months.

While none of these studies utilized a randomized control group, the convergence of findings from these five outcome studies strongly supports the concept that flower essences may be used adjunctively to facilitate the resolution of mild to moderate depression.

Depression and its Treatment

It is known that the lifetime risk for major depressive disorder is 7 to 12% for men and 20 to 25% for women (Rush, 1993a). While the range of depression may vary from mild to severe, in general, depression may be said to decrease the overall quality and productivity of life. For example, clinical samples of patients with major depressive disorder provide evidence of severe impairment in interpersonal and occupational functioning, including loss of work time (Wells et al., 1989). Patients with major depressive disorder have more physical illnesses than do other patients seen in primary care settings (Coulehan et al., 1990). And, health care utilization is increased in persons in the community with major depressive disorder compared to other patients in the general medical setting (Regier et al., 1988).

Once identified, depression can often be treated successfully with medication, psychotherapy, or a combination of both (Rush et al., 1993b). Not all patients respond to the same therapy, but a patient who fails to respond to the first treatment attempted is highly likely to respond to a different treatment. Formal treatments for major depressive disorder fall into six broad domains: medication, psychotherapy, the combination of medication and psychotherapy, electroconvulsive therapy (ECT), light therapy, and alternative therapies such as herbs and homeopathy. Each domain has benefits and risks, which must be weighed carefully in selecting the optimal treatment for a given patient.

The efficacy of the treatment of depression has been studied extensively. Rush (1993b) conducted an exhaustive review of the literature and presents the complexities of trying to monitor treatment outcomes, along with "meta-analyses" of several forms of therapy. In one such meta-analysis, 24 randomized control trials across 10 different anti-depressant medications indicated that 57.8% of the patients responded to anti-depressant medications, compared to 35.6% responding to placebos.

Today, more and more individuals are seeking non-pharmacological (alternative therapy) solutions to physical and mental disorders. Eisenberg et al. (1993), conducted a national survey indicating that one in three respondents used at least one alternative therapy in the last year, and that a third of those saw their alternative provider an average of 19 times. Similar international studies estimate that from 70 to 90% of healthcare is rendered by alternative practitioners (Micozzi, 1996). The nature of the studies presented in this article focuses upon the use of flower essence therapy, one alternative therapy, in the treatment of mild to moderate depression.

Mariposa Lily (Calochortus leichtlinii)
for disturbances in mother-child bonding

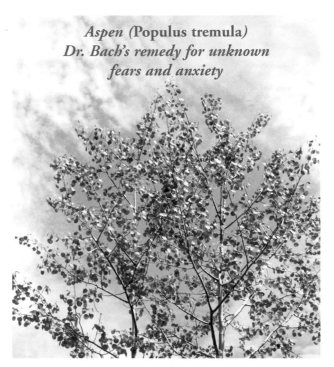

Aspen (Populus tremula)
Dr. Bach's remedy for unknown
fears and anxiety

> *Suffering is an opportunity to bring to awareness spiritual and emotional conflicts that need to be resolved so that one can fulfill his or her full potential and destiny in life.*

Flower Essence Therapy: Treating the Individual, Not the Disease

The therapeutic use of flower essence therapy in the treatment of depression and other psychologically based disorders is not new. Flower essence therapy was introduced by the English physician, Dr. Edward Bach, in the 1930s (Bach, 1931; Weeks, 1940; Barnard, 1994). Bach observed the effects of worry, anxiety, fear, confusion, indecision, depression, despair, jealousy, resentment, and the like on the health of his patients. The 38 flower remedies that he developed each address specific emotional states. Yet, Dr. Bach did not conceive of flower essence therapy as merely a means to remove emotional pain. In his book *Heal Thyself*, Dr. Bach (1931) writes that suffering is a means by which one can change. Suffering is an opportunity to bring to awareness spiritual and emotional conflicts that need to be resolved so that one can fulfill his or her full potential and destiny in life.

> *It is more important to know what sort of person has a disease than to know what sort of disease a person has. — Hippocrates*

The practitioner considers the emotional, mental, physical, and spiritual aspects (or bodies) of the individual. There is not one standard flower essence or flower essence combination that is ideally suited for treating depression. Instead, the practitioner must treat the individual, rather than the disease, selecting the particular flower essence combination that will empower the individual to change. The essences are seen as catalysts for self-awareness and change. To be successful, rather than directly treating the depression, the essence combination for the individual must awaken the energetic qualities in the individual that are out of balance or suppressed.

Prior Clinical Research in Flower Essence Therapy

Most of the clinical research on flower essences has entailed anecdotal case reports. There has been very little formal research on the topic. In conducting a deep review of the literature, it appears that only three formal studies have been conducted on the therapeutic effects of flower essences. Campanini (1997) evaluated patients before and after a flower essence treatment program of three or four months for the treatment of symptoms of anxiety, stress, and depression. Improvement was noted in 89% of patients, especially those with anxiety symptoms. An analysis of the patients' initial trust or skepticism about the treatment did not show any influence on the outcome of the treatment. Cram (2001a) utilized a randomized placebo control design to determine the influence of Bach's "emergency combination" (Five-Flower Formula) on a psychological (Paced Serial Arithmetic Task) stress response. From this study, the flower essences were noted to significantly attenuate physiological arousal compared to the placebo control. Cram (2001a) also explored the influence of the Five-Flower Formula versus the Yarrow Special Formula (currently available as Yarrow Environmental Solution) against a placebo control group on a physically stimulated (high-intensity light) stress response on QEEG and muscle tension at the sites of the chakras. From this study, it was observed that only the placebo group showed increased activation of beta activity in the frontal lobes along with increased muscular activation in the mid-back (heart) area during intense photic stimulation. Neither flower essence combination group evidenced these two stress responses. Lastly, there have been two dissertations involving flower essences (Ruhle, 1994; Weisglas, 1979), one assessing the impact of flower essences on pregnancy and the other looking at personal growth.

Flower Essence Therapy in Cuba

The emergence of flower essence therapy and the associated research in Cuba is particularly significant. With the fall of the Soviet Union and consequent ending of economic support, and the longstanding economic embargo by the United States, by 1995, Cuba was faced with an unstable economy, along with a scarcity of medical supplies and pharmaceuticals. Because of the perceived efficacy and growing worldwide interest in holistic medicine, the Cuban government mandated the establishment and integration of natural and traditional medicine into their conventional medicine national health system (MINSAP, 1996). Miyar (2002) has provided a complete description of the revolution of political and healthcare policy that led to educating healthcare practitioners in the use of flower essences as the mainline treatment of mental and emotional disorders. (See page 74 for an article by Dr. Miyar on flower essence therapy in Cuba.) The systematic evaluation of the clinical effects of flower essence therapy in the treatment of depression in Cuba was stimulated by the previous research summarized in the preliminary findings of Cram (2001b).

In this article, a series of clinical outcome studies is presented that examine the clinical efficacy of flower essence therapy as an adjunctive in the treatment of mild to moderate severity in major depression. Four new, and one prior (Cram, 2001b), clinical outcome studies are presented in this article.

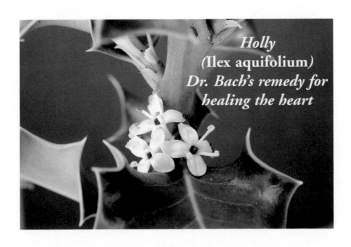

Holly
(Ilex aquifolium)
Dr. Bach's remedy for
healing the heart

A Time-Series Design Using the Beck and Hamilton Scales

The experimental design for all five studies is best described as a "quasi-experimental" time series design (Campbell & Stanley, 1963). Such a design was used extensively in 19th century experimentation for the physical and biological sciences. Its weakness, of course, is the lack of a randomized control group. However, in the behavioral sciences, simple outcome studies provide a stronger basis of information compared to single case reports. In addition, the "within subject" designs have commonly been used in initial clinical outcome studies. The statistical analysis used in all four studies consisted of a repeated measures design to account for the fact that the data set is related.

In all of the studies, the impact of the flower essences on depression was measured on two objective standard depression inventories, the Beck Depression Inventory (BDI) and the Hamilton Depression Scale (HAM-D) (Beck, 1961; Hamilton, 1968). The former is a self assessment by the patient, while the latter is a structured clinical assessment by the therapist or physician.

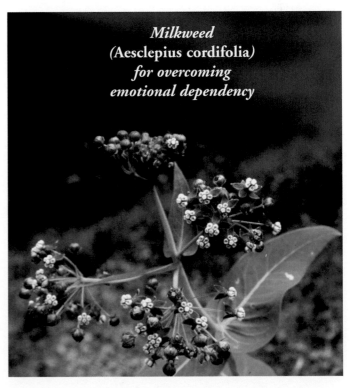

Milkweed
(Aesclepius cordifolia)
for overcoming
emotional dependency

Study 1: The Sastriques Study: At the Outpatient Clinic of the Psychiatric Hospital of Havana

The first study was completed by Dr. Pedro Sastriques Silva. (See profile on page 83). The study took place at the outpatient clinic of the Center for Specialized Treatments (DTE) at the Psychiatric Hospital of Havana, Cuba. Dr. Sastriques and three other doctors treat approximately 60 patients per week at the clinic. Twenty-three patients were selected who did not have previous treatment with flower essences, and who were suffering from depression. The method of selection was a technique of kinesiological testing by arm reflex, developed by Dr. Sastriques and his wife, Dr. Xonia Lopez. The method is known as EEI (Evaluación Enérgetica Integrativa — Integrative Energetic Evaluation.) (Sastriques 2000, 2004).

All 23 patients completed three months of flower essence therapy, most with four monthly Beck and Hamilton tests. The patients included 13 females and 10 males, ranging in age from 22 to 64, with an average age of 43. Of the 23 subjects, BDI and HAM-D data were complete for all four months for 20 subjects. There was an average of 5.2 essences selected in each session, and a total of 113 unique essences were used in the study. The twenty most frequently used essences were **Agrimony, Scleranthus, Saguaro, Crab Apple, Olive, Oak, Borage, Mimulus, Impatiens, Holly, Gentian, Chestnut Bud, White Chestnut, Mountain Pride, Chicory, Rock Water, Self-Heal, Wild Rose, Aspen** and **Pomegranate**.

The effects of flower essence therapy on both the Beck Depression Inventory ($F_{(3,57)}=142.74$; $p<.0000$) and Hamilton Depression Scale ($F_{(3,57)}=175.07$; $p<.0000$) were highly significant. Figures 1 & 2 show the significant declines in both the BDI and HAM-D scores. The BDI scores indicate that the group started out in the moderately depressed range at baseline, and ended in the "normal" range by the third month of flower essence therapy. The HAM-D scores reflect a moderate level of depression at baseline, shifting to mild levels of depression by the end of flower essence therapy.

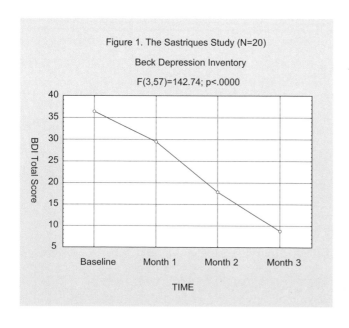

Figure 1. The Sastriques Study (N=20)

Beck Depression Inventory

$F_{(3,57)}=142.74$; $p<.0000$

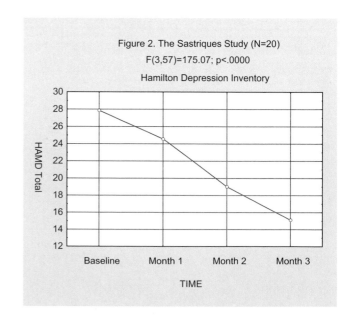

Figure 2. The Sastriques Study (N=20)

$F_{(3,57)}=175.07$; $p<.0000$

Hamilton Depression Inventory

Study 2: The Ramos Study: An Active Practice of a Cuban Psychologist

This study was conducted in Cuba by Lic. Elvira Haydée Ramos González, a psychologist at the Psychiatry Department of the Hospital and Medical Institute "Calixto García," in Havana, Cuba. (See profile on page 85.)

One hundred and nine patients were offered flower essence therapy for their depression. Fifty-four patients, representing 49.5% of the sample, completed therapy, 19 patients were still undergoing therapy at last report. Thirty-five patients abandoned therapy, and one patient died. The overall drop-out rate was 33%. The original sample consisted of 79 females and 30 males. The average age of the population was 47.4, ranging from 17 to 81 years. Patients were selected according to the criteria of the study: having had no previous flower essence therapy, reporting that they were depressed, and a willingness to volunteer for the study. Of the 54 completing the study, Hamilton Depression Scores were completed less often, with baseline and first month data available on all subjects with only 50 HAM-D assessments being conducted at the 5th month of therapy.

Individual prescribing procedures were utilized, based on a clinical interview with the patient. The 54 patients were seen monthly over the course of their therapy, for a total of 5 visits. An average of 3.2 flower essences were used in each session, out of a total of 98 unique essences. The twenty most frequently used essences were **Mariposa Lily, Dandelion, Beech, Sunflower, Lavender, Garlic, Holly, Manzanita, Chamomile, Self-Heal, Chicory, Saint John's Wort, Snapdragon, Angelica, Crab Apple, Saguaro, Yerba Santa, Forget-Me-Not, Willow,** and **California Wild Rose**.

The results of the Ramos study are presented in Figures 3 and 4 below. As can be seen in the BDI scores, there is a highly significant change in BDI scores ($F_{(4,148)}=83.54$; $p<0.000$). Here, the baseline for the depressed patients began in the high end of the severely depressed range, falling nearly 50% and into the bottom end of the moderately depressed range at the end of 4 months of flower essence therapy. Post hoc analysis, (Tukey's HSD, Tukey, 1992) shows a significant decrease in depression scores for each month compared to the prior month. The HAM-D ratings by the prescribing physician also show severe levels of depression at baseline, with a highly significant decrease in depression ($F_{(2,98)}=282.52$; $p<0.000$) being observed over the course of the 4 months. Here, there is a 66% decrease in the HAM-D scores from severely depressed at baseline to mildly depressed at month 4. Post hoc analysis (Tukey's HSD) showed significant drops for each time period.

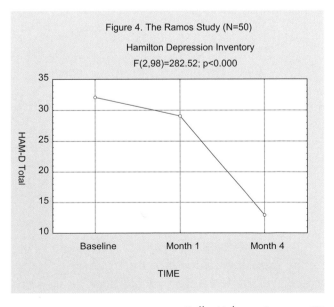

Figure 3. The Ramos Study (N=54)

Beck Depression Inventory

$F_{(4,148)}=83.54$; $p<0.000$

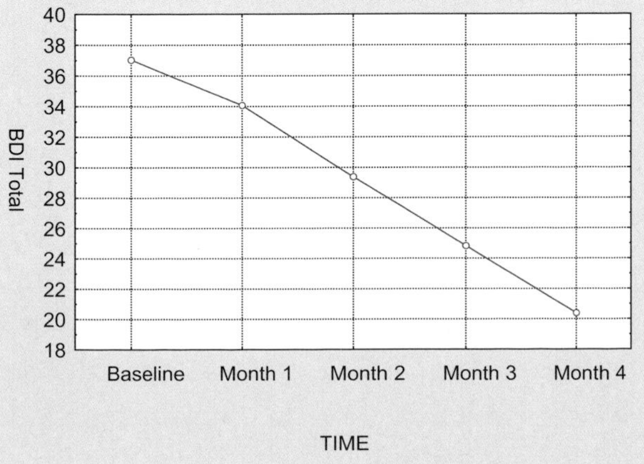

Figure 4. The Ramos Study (N=50)

Hamilton Depression Inventory

$F_{(2,98)}=282.52$; $p<0.000$

Oceans

*I have a feeling that my boat
has struck, down there in the depths,
against a great thing.*

*And nothing
Happens! Nothing…Silence…Waves…*

*—Nothing happens? Or has everything happened,
and we are standing now, quietly, in the new life?*

Juan Ramon Jimenez, translated by Robert Bly

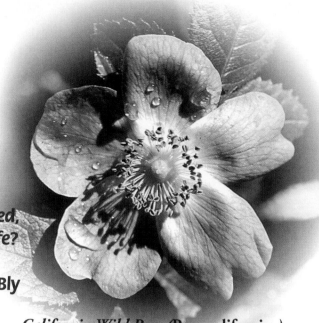

California Wild Rose (Rosa californica)
for bringing enthusiasm to life

Study 3: The de los Ángeles Study: A Psychiatric Practice in Havana

This study was conducted by Dr. María de los Ángeles Fernández de la Llera, a psychiatric physician practicing in Havana, Cuba. She has specialty degrees in Homeopathy, Traditional Chinese Medicine, Human Development and EEI (Integrative Energetic Evaluation). Dr. de los Ángeles works at the Bioenergetic and Flower Essence Therapy Department of the Psychiatric Hospital of Havana. She has participated in congresses/conferences in Bioenergetics, Natural and Traditional Medicine, and Homeopathy.

This study differs from the previous study in that more details are available about the subjects. The study consists of a pre-test and two months of treatment.

Patients were selected according to similar criteria as in the Ramos study. The selected patients had no previous flower essence therapy, reporting that they were depressed, and volunteering to be in the study.

Twenty patients were studied. All patients who entered the study completed the two-month study; there were no dropouts. The mean age of the sam-

ple was 50.12 years, ranging from 21 to 80 years. There were 4 males and 16 females. Seven of the patients had been suffering from depression for less than 1 year, with the shortest duration of depression being 3 months. The rest of the population had been suffering from depression for more than 1 year. Two had a 2-year history of depression, two had a 3-year history of depression, three had a 5-year history of depression, and one had a 6-year history of depression. Seven of the patients were concurrently on antidepressants, 9 were also utilizing tranquilizers, and 5 were concurrently receiving psychotherapy. Table 1 shows the most frequent symptoms seen in this population.

As with the prior studies, individualized prescribing was done, while using the EEI kinesiology method described previously to select flower essences for each patient. The most commonly used essences for this population were: **Mustard, Gentian, Wild Rose, Borage, Bleeding Heart, Star of Bethlehem, Sweet Chestnut, Honeysuckle, Gorse, Walnut, Chicory, Pine, Agrimony, White Chestnut, California Wild Rose, Yerba Santa, Aloe Vera, Milkweed, Sagebrush, Chamomile, Larch, Olive, Hornbeam, and Love-Lies-Bleeding**.

The results of this study are best represented in the two figures below. As can be seen in Figure 5, the BDI scores dropped significantly ($F_{(2,38)}=193.21$; $p<.0000$) from baseline through therapy. They began in the severely depressed range, reaching the normal range by month 2. Post hoc analysis (Tukey's HSD) shows significant changes for each month. In Figure 6, we see a significant decrease in HAM-D scores ($F_{(1,19)}=399.78$; $p<.0000$). Here, we see a 57% decrease in depression ratings, going from the moderately depressed, down into the mildly depressed range.

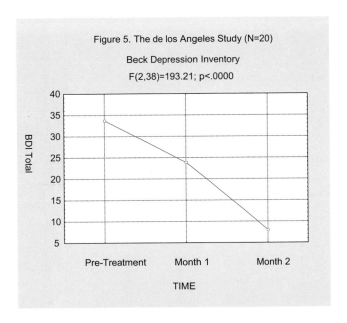

Figure 5. The de los Angeles Study (N=20)

Beck Depression Inventory

$F_{(2,38)}=193.21$; $p<.0000$

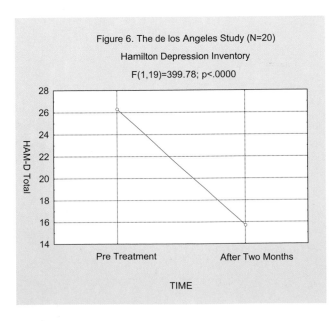

Figure 6. The de los Angeles Study (N=20)

Hamilton Depression Inventory

$F_{(1,19)}=399.78$; $p<.0000$

Table 1: The Most Common Symptoms Seen in the de los Ángeles Population		
	Female	Male
Sadness/Depression	16	4
Guilt	10	2
Sleep Disorders	16	4
Effect on Work and Leisure	11	2
Agitation	4	0
Psychic Anxiety	16	4
Somatic Anxiety	9	2
Gastrointestinal Somatic Symptoms	8	1
General Somatic Symptoms	11	3
Loss of Sex Drive	13	2
Hypochondria	4	0
Weight Loss	5	1

Study 4: The Tena Study: A Holistic Psychiatric Practice

The fourth Cuban study is by Dr. Sol Inés Tena Rodríguez, a psychiatric doctor specializing in children and youth. She has taken courses in homeopathy, and traditional Chinese medicine (acupuncture), and has earned diplomas in Homeopathy; Human Development; and EEI (Integrative Energetic Evaluation). She is a member of the national group of professors of Flower Essence Therapy.

Dr. Tena works solely with natural and traditional medicines, including flower essences, homeopathy, and acupuncture at the 26 de Julio Polyclinic, Playa Township, Havana. She has participated in various conferences in Psychiatry, Homeopathy, and Natural and Traditional Medicine.

She presented a paper on her depression study research at the Ninth International Congress of Flower Essence Therapists (IX Congreso Internacional de Terapeutas Florales) in Cuernavaca, Mexico, October, 2002. Portions of this article are based on data presented at that congress.

Dr. Tena's study provides a more complete picture of the treatment outcome effects than the other studies, and contains much descriptive data on the population studied.

Patients for the study either showed up at the clinic on their own initiative for treatment for depression, or, more frequently, were referred by other doctors from the clinic where Dr. Tena works. Individual prescribing procedures were utilized, based on a clinical interview with the patient. Three of these subjects dropped out of the study, and there was incomplete data on one subject's initial HAM-D score, leaving 24 subjects for analysis for the BDI data and 23 subjects for the HAM-D data. There were 21 females and 3 males. The mean age of the population was 54.1 years, ranging from 33 to 75 years of age. The characteristics of depression are detailed in the tables on the next page. Table 2 shows the duration of the depression, while Table 3 shows the major symptoms of the group.

A total of 65 different flower essences were used for the 28 subjects. Table 4 shows the most commonly used essences and the therapeutic conflicts they address.

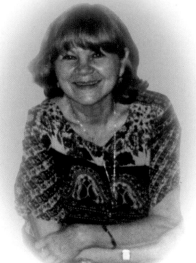

Dr. Sol Inés Tena Rodríguez

At the beginning of the study, 26 of the 28 patients were taking psycho-pharmaceutical medication. Dosages were gradually reduced and eliminated by the end of the study. Table 5 shows the drugs that were used by patients at the beginning of the study.

The outcome results of the study are presented in the two figures below. As can be seen in Figure 7, there is a significant decrease in the Beck Depression Inventory scores across time ($F(3,69)=100.21$; $p<.0000$). Here, the levels of depression go from the moderate range to the normal range. In addition, the effects of the flower essences on depression tend to stabilize by the second month of treatment. The data for the second and third months do not significantly differ, while all other comparisons are significant using Tukey's HSD. In addition, Figure 8 shows significant effects of flower essences on the Hamilton Depression Scale as well ($F(1,22)=162.59$; $p<0000$). The changes go from the severe range of depression to "nearly normal" levels of mood and affect.

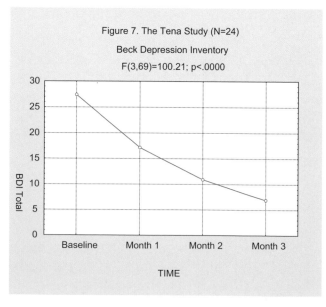

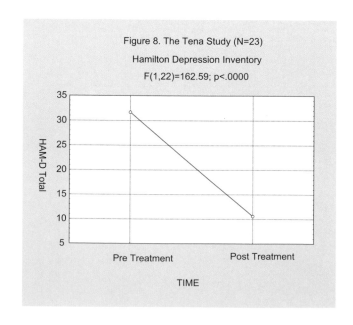

Table 2: Duration of Depression in the Tena Study

Duration	Number
1 month	3
2 months	1
3 months	6
4 months	2
5 months	2
6 months	2
10 months	1
1 year	1
2 years	2
3 years	5
25 years	1
27 years	1
Unknown	1

Table 3: Common Presenting Symptoms of the Tena Population

Symptom	Cases
Sadness	28
General Somatic Symptoms	23
Insight	23
Psychic Anxiety	23
Sleep Disorders	20
Somatic Anxiety	20
Hypochondria	18
Loss of Sex Drive	17
Guilt	16
Inhibited Speech or Thought	16
Loss of Appetite	16
Worsening of Symptoms in the Afternoon	16
Decline in Work Productivity	13
Symptoms of Obsession and Compulsion	13
Sudden Loss of Reality	11
Worsening of Symptoms in the Morning	11
Agitation	7
Suicidal Tendencies	7
Weight Loss	7
Suspect Symptoms of Paranoia	6
Other symptoms: Hopelessness, Distress, Self-aggression, Loneliness, Fear	

Table 4: Commonly Used Flower Essences in the Tena Study

Flower Essence	Therapeutic Conflict
Aloe Vera	For restoring exhausted vital energy when run down
Black-Eyed Susan	For blocking and repression, looking at the hidden side (shadow)
Bleeding Heart	For freeing from pathological and symbiotic emotional attachments
Borage	To provide joy in cases of abasement, grief, and disappointment
California Wild Rose	For dealing with apathy and lack of interest
Gentian	For reactive depression
Mountain Pride	To protect from negative thoughts and give strength to fight for life
Mustard	For endogenous depression
Self-Heal	To develop inner power of healing
Tansy	To stimulate decision to combat lack of initiative
Yarrow	For protection in midst of conflict

Table 5: Psycho-Pharmaceuticals Used by Patients at the Beginning of the Treatment in the Tena Study

Drug	Number of Cases
Trifluoperazine	9
Amitriptyline	9
Clorodiazepoxide	9
Diazepam	5
Nitrazepam	5
Imipramine	3
Medazepam	3
Meprobamate	3
Thioridazine	3

Study 5: The Cram Study: A Multi-Site Study in the USA

This is a multi-site study conducted in the United States. It has been previously published, and greater detail about the study's parameters may be seen in the original paper (Cram, 2001). In this study, a baseline of one month is collected during "usual care." Starting with the second month, the experimental treatment (flower essence therapy, described below) was added to the usual care. From a "within subject" A-B design perspective, when the baseline period is stable prior to the experimental procedure, any changes post-baseline are likely to be attributed to the experimental procedure.

There were 12 subjects in this study, coming from four clinical trial sites. The sites are listed at the bottom of Table 7. Three of the clinical trial sites were psychotherapy practices, contributing 11 of the 12 subjects to the study. Two of the psychotherapy practices were transpersonal in nature, while the third was cognitive and behavioral in its approach. The non-psychotherapy clinic was a naturopathic practice in which a combination of nutritional support was offered along with wellness counseling. There were 3 male and 9 female subjects, aged 35 to 79 years of age, with a mean of 48.5 years. They had been depressed for an average of 22 years. Nine had tried antidepressants, while 3 had not. At the time of the study, 8 patients were currently on an antidepressant, and had been on these for an average of 17 months.

Treatment was comprised of usual care, followed by usual care in combination with flower essence therapy. In all but one clinical trial site, the usual care entailed psychotherapy. One clinical trial site utilized naturopathic counseling for usual care. Over the course of the experimental treatment phase, patients were offered an average of eight different flower essences. Across the 12 subjects, a total of 65 different flower essences were used. For any given patient, the range of essences used went from a minimum of five essences for 1 patient to a maximum of 13 different essences for another patient. The flower essence therapy uti-

lized an "individualized" approach and was directed by the philosophy of "treating the individual, rather than the disease (depression)." The particular flower essence combination used with a patient was selected based upon the areas in the patient's life for which the therapist felt the patient needed support or were emerging as part of the counseling.

To give a sense of how flower essences are used clinically to treat depressed individuals in this study, the nine most common flower essences offered to these patients, along with their therapeutic themes, are listed in Table 6 (in alphabetical order). These essences occurred consistently in at least 25% of the patients.

Table 6: Therapeutic Themes of the Nine Most Commonly Used Flower Essences Used to Treat Depression in the Cram Study

Themes were abstracted from the *Flower Essence Repertory* (Kaminski & Katz, 1994).

Essence	Primary Defining Quality
Aspen	To draw upon inner strength while calming vague anxieties
Black-Eyed Susan	To awaken consciousness with penetrating insight into past traumas
California Wild Rose	To deal with apathy or resignation; to stimulate enthusiasm for life
Dandelion	To deal with tense over-striving while allowing greater inner ease and balance
Larch	To replace lack of confidence and failure with renewed self-confidence
Olive	To deal with exhaustion and fatigue by revitalizing the soul
Peppermint	To replace mental sluggishness with mindfulness and clarity
Scotch Broom	To replace pessimism and despair with optimism
Star Thistle	To replace the inability to give of oneself with a sense of abundance and trust

The results of the Cram study are presented at two levels. The first represents simple descriptive statistics on the level of change in depression for each subject, and the second analysis utilizes inferential statistics.

The descriptive statistics are presented in Table 7 below. Along with the demographic of the subject, the presence or absence of antidepressant use is described. In addition, the total number of flower essences taken by the subject over the treatment period is given, along with the number of times the clinician changed the flower essence formula over the course of the patient's care.

As can be seen in this table, one half of the subjects made substantial changes in their depression scores (Beck change scores that were 10 points or more), one third of the subjects made moderate gains, and only 2 subjects made minimal changes. One should note that there are some discrepancies between the subjects' self-ratings of depression (Beck) and those of the therapists (HAM-D). The level of change in the depression scores, however, does not appear to consistently sort along the lines of the clinical site (therapist), the use of antidepressant drugs, the total number of flower essences used to treat the patient, or the number of times the therapist changed the flower essence formula over the course of therapy.

In addition to the descriptive statistics above, two separate analyses using inferential statistics (ANOVA) were conducted. Each analysis involved an analysis of variance with repeated measures because of related samples. The first analysis considered the Period Effect. Here, the "within variable" had 5 levels (2 baseline, plus the 3 treatment measures.) In the second analysis, the interaction effects of concurrent use of antidepressants was considered. This was conducted using a group-blocking variable for current use of an antidepressant. As can be seen in Table 7, there were 8 subjects that were currently on antidepressants and 4 that were not.

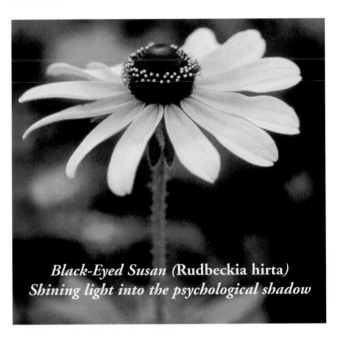

Black-Eyed Susan **(Rudbeckia hirta)**
Shining light into the psychological shadow

Table 7: Descriptive Statistics & Mean Change, Baseline to Treatment Phase, Cram Study												
Attribute/Subject no.	1	2	3	4	5	6	7	8	9	10	11	12
Age/Sex	37/M	43/F	66/F	52/F	39/F	49/F	53/F	40/F	79/M	35/F	41/F	49/M
Clinical Site	1	2	1	3	3	3	3	2	1	2	2	4
Antidepressant	Prozac	None	None	Zoloft	Prozac	Pamelar	Prozac	Effexor	None	None	Celexa	Prozac
Total number of flower essences used	5	13	7	12	9	9	11	7	5	7	6	7
Number of changes in flower essence formula	1	3	1	2	2	2	2	1	0	2	0	3
Beck Change	16.83	14.33	6.00	2.83	13.50	4.83	6.83	6.67	12.17	8.00	4.00	0.00
HAM-D Change	12.00	17.00	8.00	12.00	9.50	9.00	17.50	8.50	11.00	12.50	2.50	4.50

Clinical Sites: 1= Jeffrey R. Cram, Ph.D (Nevada City, CA); 2= Constance Rodriguez, Ph.D.(Nevada City, CA); 3= Beth Wortzel, M.A., CSW (Madison, WI); 4=Reba Hatfield, N.D. (Charlotte, NC)

The results for Period Effect are reflected in Figures 9 and 10. As can be seen, the statistics on both the Beck Depression Inventory $(F(4,40)=12.46; p<.0000)$ and Hamilton scores $(F(2,20)=22.79; p<.0000)$ are highly significant, indicating that this Period Effect is highly consistent. The post hoc analysis shows that the two baseline data points are not significantly different from each other, while the treatment data points for both the BDI and HAM-D were significantly lower than the baseline points. Overall, the depression ratings dropped by approximately 50% during the treatment phase for both the BDI and HAM-D variables. These ratings shifted from the moderately depressed range down into the lower end of the mildly depressed range.

The second analysis concerning the concurrent use of antidepressant medications ("SSRI") is presented in Figures 11 and 12. As can be seen, the level of significance for the two-way interactions (Period x Medication Group) was not significant for either the BDI $(F(4,40)=.90; p<.4752)$ or the HAM-D $(F(2,20)=.77; p<.4754)$. The decrease in both the BDI and HAM-D scores was similar, whether or not the subject was on an SSRI. This suggests that the use of anti-depressants did not interact with the effects of the flower essences, and strongly suggests that the effect on depression was solely due to the flower essences, and not the allopathic medications.

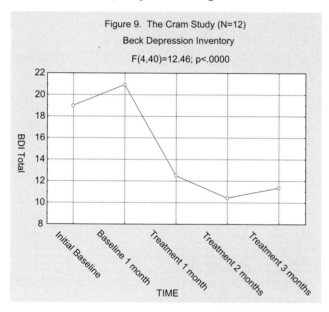

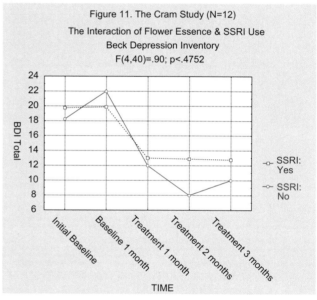

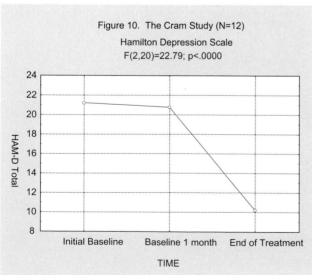

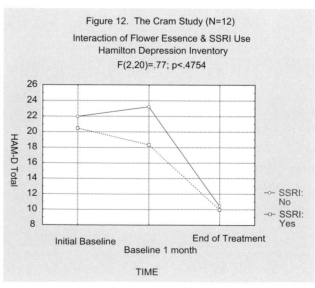

> *What is being tested in these studies is not a specific flower essence (or a specific combination of essences), but rather a method of individualized flower essence treatment.*

Discussion: Individualized Treatment

This paper presents a series of independent studies on the use of flower essences in the treatment of depression. All five independent studies represent uncontrolled outcome studies, with each providing different levels of information. All five studies show a significant decrease in depression associated with the use of flower essence therapy. Taken as a whole, there is convergent data that supports the clinical use of flower essences in the treatment of depression.

It should be noted that there are several challenges to both the internal and external validity of these current studies. The first challenge has to do with "individualized" treatment versus standardized treatment. The "individualized" prescribing method of the flower essence practitioner certainly confuses the traditional operational definition of the independent variable. In the above studies, over 100 different flower essences were utilized, with an average of eight different essences being administered to a given subject. What is being tested in these studies is not a specific flower essence (or a specific combination of essences), but rather a method of individualized flower essence treatment. Such an "individualized" approach of "treating the individual, rather than the disease," is very common in homeopathy. A recent meta-analysis by Cucherat et al. (2000) examined 118 clinical trials that involved individualized homeopathic therapies, and a slightly earlier meta-analysis by Linde and Melchart (1998) examined 32 clinical trials that compared individualized homeopathic therapies to placebo controls. While such an individualized prescribing approach does lend "noise" to the independent variable and the scientific method, it is the clinical method of choice for the alternative practitioner who uses flower essences, and thus should be allowed as a valid method.

Considering the Placebo Effect

The second threat to the internal validity of the study is its lack of a randomized control procedure. Without such controls, we cannot exclude the possible contamination to the study due to history, maturation, selection bias, and the placebo effect. One could cogently argue, for example, that the decrease in the depression scores had nothing to do with flower essences at all, but were merely a reflection of the sincerity and increased enthusiasm of the practitioner as he or she introduces the flower essences into the treatment of the patient.

However, in previous unpublished research on the use of flower essences on the treatment of depression, the senior author has conducted a pilot study on 6 subjects that employed a randomized double-blind placebo control group design. In this study, all 3 of the experimental subjects (flower essence) responded in the same fashion as did the subjects in the current study, with large, 50% or more, decrements in their BDI scores. In addition, 2 of the 3 placebo subjects (brandy carrier only) showed an impressive 50% decrement in BDI scores during the first month of

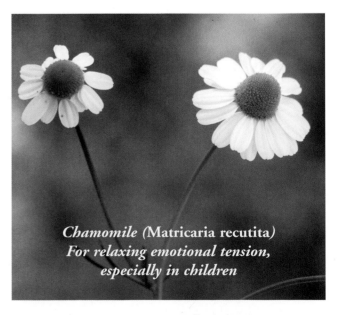

Chamomile (Matricaria recutita)
For relaxing emotional tension, especially in children

treatment. However, by the second month of treatment, the BDI scores of the placebo responders were back to baseline and stayed elevated into the third month of placebo treatment. One of the placebo subjects was converted into a single case study format, and at the beginning of month 4, she was given the authentic individualized flower essence therapy. By the end of month 4, her BDI scores were reduced by 50% again. This time the BDI stayed down for the next 2 months. Such a crossover single subject design is very attractive, and lends evidence to the effectiveness of flower essences in the treatment of depression. Unfortunately, it is difficult to generalize beyond this one subject. It was the lack of generalization associated with single-subject designs that was the primary reason for the selection of the time series/within subject design used in the above studies.

The problem with the placebo effect is not the fact that it exists. We should all celebrate its existence. The problem with the placebo effect is that its effects are typically short-lived and small in nature. Recent evidence suggests that patients with different types of depression and prognoses react differently to placebo and treatment. Schatzberg and Rothschild (in press) reported that the placebo response rate for nonpsychotic major depressive disorder is on the order of 25%, while the placebo response rate for psychotic depressions is only about 10%. The outcomes of the current study were in the 50% range, and far exceed those solely attributable to the placebo response.

Next, consider the duration of the placebo effect. Its therapeutic effects are typically short-lived, lasting 2 to 4 weeks. In the Cram and Tena studies, the 3-month treatment period is one of

the strongest arguments in favor of the fact that flower essences were more active than the placebo effect. This is reflected in the fact that the changes in the BDI and HAM-D scores endured over a 3-month period of time.

Some might argue that depression typically resolves more slowly than over a period of 4 months, and that that is why most studies of depression span a period of 6 to 9 months. The 2- to 4-month nature of the current studies may not allow one to examine the true nature of the treatment response. Some patients, for example, may relapse after the initial reprieve, while others may not respond to the treatment until the fifth or sixth month. The 4-month duration of the current study lacks follow-up and the possible assessment of relapse. Thus, the short duration of these studies may possibly weaken their findings.

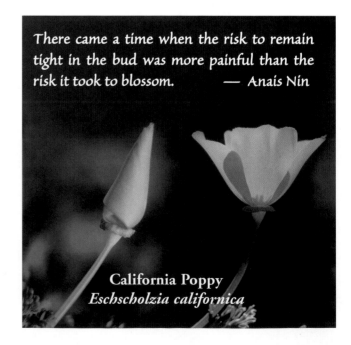

There came a time when the risk to remain tight in the bud was more painful than the risk it took to blossom.   — Anais Nin

California Poppy
Eschscholzia californica

A secondary analysis of the data by Cram was conducted to determine whether SSRI medications would interfere with the therapeutic use of flower essences, and vice versa. This post hoc analysis did not show a separation between the two groups (SSRI medicated and unmedicated) in their responses to the introduction of flower essence therapy. Thus, it appears that being on an SSRI does not interfere with the psychotherapeutic and flower essence aspects of the treatment. One should note, however, that the small number of patients in the medicated and unmedicated groups, coupled with their self-selection, weakens our ability to generalize the results to the population in general.

The fact that we see such significant response curves to the use of flower essences in all five studies clearly suggests that practitioners can use non-toxic, energetic substances to assist their patients in coping more effectively with depression. In a psychotherapy practice, flower essences appear to provide the practitioner with a tool to assist the patient in resolving psychological issues that pertain to and perpetuate depression. Some practitioners might think of a flower essence remedy as a "transitional object" (Winnicott, 1953). For example, during the psychotherapy session, the therapist might be assisting the patient to become more aware of how the patient's traumatic childhood plays a role in her chronic depression. As part of the therapy, the practitioner adds Black-Eyed Susan to the flower essence combination and tells the patient that this will assist her in retrieving or resolving those childhood memories. The theme, initiated during the therapeutic session, is facilitated and continued at home by the patient through her use of the essence. The flower essences reinvigorate the theme as they are taken orally on a daily basis.

The large number of replications presented in this paper document the clinical effectiveness of flower essences in the treatment of depression and provide a strong and compelling basis for using these tools clinically to treat depression. Further inquiry is, of course, needed. Randomized control group studies would provide additional evidence, along with longer, 6- to 8-month periods of treatment. Ultimately, randomized placebo-controlled studies would provide the strongest base of evidence as to the effectiveness of these nontoxic flower essences in the treatment of depression.

Dr. Jeffrey Cram, Ph.D. is currently the director of the Sierra Health Institute of Nevada City, California, where he coordinates and treats patients using a holistic approach to psychology. This includes such approaches as transpersonal psychology, cognitive behavioral therapies, biofeedback, flower essence therapy, aromatherapy, bioenergetics and music therapy. He is the founding president of the Surface EMG Society of North America (SESNA). He is the author of three books and 35 articles on surface Electromyography, has an active interest in research, and is currently the Principal Investigator on a Flower Essence and Depression clinical trial, and is consulting on several clinical studies. He is on the editorial list of four journals (AJPM, JAPB, JMPT, IJHC). Dr. Cram is an international expert on surface Electromyography and the use of flower essences in a psychotherapeutic practice.

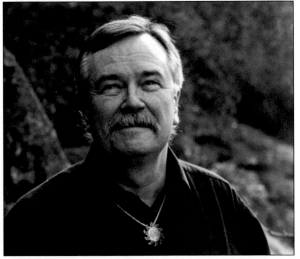

Contact information:
Dr. Jeffrey Cram, Ph.D., Sierra Health Institute
202 Providence Mine Rd., Suite 202
Nevada City, CA 95959 USA
phone: (530) 478-9660, fax: (530) 478-1432
e-mail: cram@semg.org website: www.semg.org

References

Bach, E. (1931). *Heal Thyself.* Essex, England: C.W. Daniel.

Barnard, J. (Ed.). (1994). *Collected Writings of Edward Bach.* Bath, England: Ashgrove Press.

Barnard, J., & Barnard, M. (1994). *The Healing Herbs of Edward Bach: An illustrated guide to the flower remedies.* Bath, England: Ashgrove Press.

Beck, A. T., Ward, C. H., Mendelson, M., Mock, J., & Erbaugh, J. (1961). An inventory for measuring depression. *Archives of General Psychiatry, 4,* 561-571.

Campanini, M. (1997). Bach flower therapy: Results of a monitored study of 115 patients. *La Medicina Biologica* (Italy), 15(2), 1-13.

Campbell, D., & Stanley, J. (1963). *Experimental and quasi-experimental designs for research.* Chicago: Rand-McNally.

Cram, J. R. (2000). A psychological and metaphysical study of Dr. Edward Bach's flower essence stress formula. *Subtle Energies and Energy Medicine Journal,* Volume 11, No. 1.

Cram, J. R. (2001a). Effects of two flower essences on high intensity environmental stimulation and EMF. *Subtle Energies and Energy Medicine Journal,* Volume 12, No. 3.

Cram, J. R. (2001b) "Flower Essence Therapy in the Treatment of Major Depression: Preliminary Findings" *International Journal of Healing and Caring,* Volume 1, No. 1, published on-line at http://www.ijhc.org/FreeJournal/Journal/0601articles/Cram-I-1.asp Portions of this article are taken from the IJHC article.

Coulehan, J. L., Schulberg, H. C., Block, M. R., Janosky, J. E., & Arena, V. C. (1990). Medical co-morbidity of major depressive disorder in a primary medical practice. *Archives of Internal Medicine, 150,* 2363-2367.

Cucherat, M., Haugh, M. C., Gooch, M., & Boissel, J. P. (2000). Evidence of clinical efficacy of homeopathy: A meta-analysis of clinical trials. Homeopathic Medicines Research Advisory Group. *European Journal of Clinical Pharmacology, 56*(1), 27-33.

Eisenberg, D. M., Kessler, R. C., Foster, C., Norlock, F. E., Calkins, D. R., & Delbanco, T. L. (1993). Unconventional medicine in the United States: Prevalence, costs, and patterns of use. *New England Journal of Medicine,* 328:(4), 246-252.

Gerber, R. (1988). *Vibrational medicine: New choices for healing ourselves.* Santa Fe, NM: Bear.

Hamilton, M. (1968). Development of a rating scale for primary depressive illness. *British Journal of Social Clinical Psychology, 6*(2), 78-96.

Kaminski, P. (1998). *Flowers that Heal: How to use flower essences.* Dublin, Ireland: Gill & Macmillan.

Kaminski, P., & Katz, R. (1994, 1996). *Flower Essence Repertory.* Nevada City, CA: Flower Essence Society.

Kramer D. (1995). *New Bach Flower Therapies.* Rochester, NY: Healing Arts Press.

Ministerio de Salud Pública (MINSAP) (Ministry of Public Health). (1996). Programa nacional para el desarrollo y generalización de la medicina natural y tradicional (National program for the development of natural and traditional medicine). Havana, Cuba: MINSAP.

Miyar, Beatriz M., Ph.D. (2002). *Continuing education in cuban healthcare: holistic medicine and flower essence therapy.* Doctoral dissertation. Florida State University, Tallahassee, Florida.

Linde, K., & Melchart, D. (1998). Randomized controlled trials of individualized homeopathy: A state-of-the-art review. *Journal of Alternative & Complementary Medicine, 4*(4), 371-388.

Micozzi, M. (Ed). (1996). *Fundamentals of complementary and alternative medicine.* New York: Churchill Livingstone.

Regier, D. A., Hirschfeld, M. A., Goodwin, F. K., Burke J. D., Lazar, J. B., Judd, L. (1988). The NIMH depression awareness, recognition and treatment program: structure, aims and scientific basis. *The American Journal of Psychiatry,* 145:1351-7.

Rühle, G. (1994). Pilot study on the use of Bach Flower Essences in primiparae with postdate pregnancy. Dissertation. Heidelberg University Hospital for Women, and Institute of Psychology, Tübingen (Germany).

Rush, J. A. (Chairman). (1993a). *Depression Guideline Panel. Depression in primary care: Volume 1: Detection and diagnosis. Clinical Practice Guideline, Number 5.* (AHCPR Publication No. 93-0550). Rockville, MD: U.S. Department of Health and Human Services, Public Health Service, Agency for Health Care Policy and Research.

Rush, J. A. (Chairman). (1993b). *Depression Guideline Panel. Depression in primary care: Volume 2: Treatment of major depression. Clinical Practice Guideline, Number 5.* (AHCPR Publication No. 93-0551). Rockville, MD: U.S. Department of Health and Human Services, Public Health Service, Agency for Health Care Policy and Research.

Sastriques (2000), P., Lopez, X., and Am, Elsa, *Un Viaje al Reino de la Metáfora* (A Voyage to the Realm of Metaphor) Editorial Pandemia: Argentina: description of DEI (Diagnóstico Energético Integral — Integral Energetic Diagnosis), now known as EEI (Evaluación Enérgetica Integrativa — Integrative Energetic Evaluation).

Sastriques, P. (2004). *La experiencia cubana para una medicina integrativa: la Evaluación Energética Integrativa,*(The Cuban Experience of an Integreative Medicine: Integrative Energetic Evaluation), presented at Congreso Internacional de Terapias Bioenergéticas, Tarragona, Spain, March 12-13, 2004. Universidad Rovira i Virgili. Available (in Spanish) from the Flower Essence Society.

Schatzberg, A. F., and Rothschild, A. J. (In press). Psychotic (delusional) major depression: Issues for DSM-IV. In A. J. Frances & T. Widiger (Eds.), *DSM-IV sourcebook.* Washington, DC: American Psychiatric Press.

Scheffer, M. (1986). *Bach Flower Therapy.* Wellingsborough, England: Thorsons.

Scheffer, M. (1996). *Mastering Bach Flower Therapy: A guide to diagnosis and treatment.* Rochester, NY: Healing Arts Press.

Selye, H. (1956). *The Stress of Life.* New York: McGraw-Hill.

Tukey, John (1992). *Collected Works of John Tukey: Factorial and ANOVA,* Boca Raton, FL: CRC Press.

Weisglas, M. (1979). *Personal growth and conscious evolution through Bach flower essences.* Dissertation. California Institute of Asian Studies (currently named the California Institute of Integral Studies).

Weissman, M. M. (1979). The psychological treatment of depression: Evidence for the efficacy of psychotherapy alone, and in comparison with, and in combination with pharmacotherapy. *Archives of General Psychiatry, 36,* 1261-1269.

Weissman, M. M., Klerman, G. L., Prusoff., B. A., Sholomskas, D., & Padian, N. (1981). Depressed outpatients: Results one year after treatment with drugs and/or interpersonal psychotherapy. *Archives of General Psychiatry, 38,* 51-55.

Weeks, N. (1940). *The Medical Discoveries of Edward Bach, Physician.* Essex, England: C.W. Daniel.

Wells, K. B., Stewart, A., Hays, R. D., Burnam, M. A., Rogers, W., Daniels M., et al. (1989). The functioning and well-being of depressed patients: Results from the Medical Outcomes Study. *The Journal of the American Medical Association, 262*(7), 914-919.

Winnicott, D. (1953). Transitional objects and transitional phenomena. *International Journal of Psychoanalysis,* 34, 89-97.

Wright, M. S. (1988). *Flower Essences: Reordering our understanding and approach to illness and health.* Warrenton, VA: Perelandra.

Flower Essences for Mid-Life Crisis in Women: A Pilot Study in Mexico

Elizabeth Heyns, Psychologist

Abstract

Aims:

☆ Pilot study to assess anxiety, depression, physical symptoms and flower essence needs in perimenopausal-aged women.

☆ Describe the most-needed flower essences at the time of the study as related to the most commonly affected areas of subjects' lives.

☆ Evaluate the effectiveness of the Zung Scale for Depression, the Rojas Scale for Anxiety, and the Questionnaire of Physical Symptoms (Heyns), and decide whether they are to be used as-is, changed, or replaced in the central research.

Design:

Quasi-experimental study with intervention (flower essence therapy).

Location:

Private practice in Tepoztlán, Morelos Province, and Mexico City, Mexico

Population and sample:

Ten women between 40 and 55 years of age (mean: 46.5, median: 45.5); non-probabilistic sample with voluntary subjects.

Intervention:

Six sessions were conducted, once per month. During the first and last sessions, subjects were evaluated for traits of depression (Zung Scale for Depression), anxiety (Rojas Scale for Anxiety), physical symptoms of menopause, and specific needs for flower essences (Client Background Information intake form provided by the *Flower Essence Society*). Subjects were treated with flower essences, which were defined during each session.

Results:

There was a general reduction of symptoms, anxiety, and depression. Depression was reduced by 28%, with a final value of "normal" as defined by Zung. Anxiety was reduced 42% in the variety and quantity of anxiety situations, 28% in the intensity of anxiety felt, with a final level of 18% on the Rojas scale, considered as a "normal" value. Physical symptoms were also reduced. Subjects also increased their knowledge of menopause and of themselves, deciding to continue with flower essence therapy in order to increase their capacity to deal with negative and painful emotions, improve their self-image and feelings about themselves, reduce stress, enhance their creativity and self-expression, have a greater spiritual awareness, and bring a more positive attitude toward life.

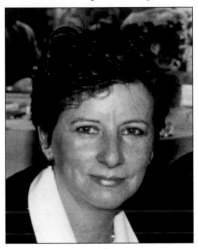

Elizabeth Heyns is a psychologist and psychotherapist who has included flower essences in her practice since 1996. She has a psychoanalytic background, but her present trend is toward the humanistic way of thought, reflecting her training as a psychotherapist in Gestalt Therapy. She also has training in couples and family therapy, and works with EMDR (Eye Movement Desensitization and Reprocessing), body memories, and TPA (Tapas) energetic change of patterns.

Elizabeth studied flower essence therapy with Barbara Espeche in 1996 and attended the FES Practitioner Training Program in 2002. She received certification from the *Flower Essence Society* in November, 2003. She has attended international symposia and flower essence congresses, at which she has presented papers on menopause.

Elizabeth's professional speciality includes menopausal transition for women and couples' relations. Elizabeth is currently living in Spain. She can be contacted by writing to Elizabeth Heyns, Casanova 14 2O. 2A. Der., Barcelona, 08011, Spain, or e-mail to eheyns@hotmail.com

Introduction

Midlife crisis affects both men and women, but it is more evident in women, in whom menopause is expressed in a wide range of physical symptoms.

Women deal with menopause in different ways: among others, by using HRT (Hormonal Replacement Therapy) or dietary supplements and natural remedies. But a menopausal woman deals not only with physical changes; at this point in her life she is going through a wide range of experiences. She may be dealing with issues surrounding her partner (if she has one), children (most likely adolescents or young adults who are beginning to leave home, resulting in the "empty nest" syndrome), parents (who are likely older, perhaps in need of care or facing terminal illness), and work, which she may be resuming again after years as a homemaker, or, perhaps she has been working for many years in addition to being a mother, housewife and wife — resulting in being a "tired superwoman." Finally, she encounters in midlife, an existential crisis — Who am I? What have I accomplished? And what am I going to do with the rest of my life?

Finally, she encounters in midlife, an existential crisis — Who am I? What have I accomplished? And what am I going to do with the rest of my life?

Basically, until now, this kind of crisis has been resolved solely as a physical "menopause" issue, leaving aside the many emotional aspects the woman goes through.

Flower essence therapy is a holistic therapy that primarily addresses emotional symptoms, but has an effect on physical symptoms as well. It has been found to be very useful in times of crisis. Flower essence therapy has been used for more than 70 years, and is well-known as part of natural, complementary, and/or alternative medicine.

The basic goal of this research is to show that flower essence therapy, when used successfully, can treat the emotional symptoms of the midlife woman, reducing or eliminating physical symptoms, reducing feelings of depression and anxiety, encouraging the will to know more about herself, enhancing her personal growth, and preparing her for a more fulfilling "golden age."

Subjects and Methods

Ten midlife women were treated for six months, once per month, with flower essences.

The women were searching for therapeutic help to solve issues related to family, work, health, and general welfare.

They all took part in the research voluntarily.

During the first session, they were asked to write an autobiography. They were also asked to fill out a socio-demographic questionnaire, the Zung Scale for Depression, the Rojas Scale for Anxiety, a questionnaire on physical symptoms, a clinical history of their health and sexuality, and the *Flower Essence Society* "Client Background Information" form.

All of the women were between the ages of 40 and 55 (mean: 46.5, median: 45.5). The mean number of children was 1.5 per woman (mean age: 15.5, with a proportion of nearly two girls per boy). One subject was a widow, three were single, and six were married. All were from middle-class homes. Four worked full-time, three half-time, two part-time or occasionally, and one did not work. Four took care of 100 percent of the family expenses, two were responsible for 50 percent, and three for 25 percent. The family income of three of the women was less than $1,000 U.S. per month, four had an income of less than $3,000 U.S. per month, and three received more than $3,000 U.S. per month. Seven of the women had a university degree, and others had some other type of professional background.[1]

Results of the health and sexual history questionnaire were as follows: three were still menstruating, one had a hysterectomy done during the study, five were menstruating irregularly, and one was no longer menstruating. Most of the women had learned about menstruation at school or from friends. Half the women reported feeling "normal" when menstruation first appeared, with three reported feeling scared or afraid. Today they are more open with their daughters, all reporting that they talk about this issue and about sexuality openly with them. Four of the women reported not taking anything for menopause, four reported taking natural remedies, and two reported taking HRT.

The psychological area was the most affected negatively, which shows that emotional and affective issues were more intensely felt.

Almost none of the women reported working out regularly. Half of them had both a Pap smear and a mammogram test conducted more than two years previously. Only four had ever had a hormonal profile and a densitometry test, two of these within the previous year.

During each session, notes were taken on the significant events in the women's lives, as well as on the flower essences taken and their results.

During the last session, the women were again asked to fill out the tests on depression and anxiety, the questionnaire on physical symptoms, and their reasons for taking flower essences.

Results

Rojas Anxiety Test

The general results showed a reduction of anxiety.

The intellectual area was the most affected at the beginning of the study, probably because most of the women had university or professional training which had not been utilized during the past 15 years.

The physical area was one of the least affected negatively. This sustains the hypothesis that women suffer more at this stage from emotional distress than from physical symptoms.

In terms of intensity, the psychological area was the most affected negatively, which shows that emotional and affective issues were more intensely felt.

In the last evaluation, the changes showed an anxiety decrease in all areas.

In terms of the quantity of anxiety aspects (indicated as "items"), the general reduction was 28 percent; in terms of intensity, the reduction was 42 percent. The Rojas proportional grade reduction was 18 percent.

The most important physical problem that affected the women was a decline in sexual interest. In the psychological area, sadness, melancholy, and even the feeling of "void" were present; in the behavioral area, they complained of low performance, tension (particularly in the jaw), and a feeling of mental blockage or not knowing what to say or do; in the intellectual area, the most outstanding items had to do with memory, attention, and the difficulty of concentrating; in the assertive area, they appeared to feel more comfortable alone than with strangers.

The graph below shows the proportional reduction for each area.

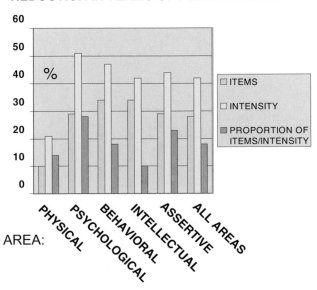

GENERAL RESULTS OF THE ANXIETY TEST: REDUCTION IN TERMS OF PERCENTAGES

Zung Depression Scale

Using the Zung Self-Rating Depression Scale (SDS) as a measure, the study found that in general, depression decreased by 28 percent. Only one woman did not show a decrease in depression. She was the oldest of the group, who had already passed menopause several years before, and had a normal depression score. All others ended the study within the "normal" range.

In terms of the specific depression issues, the ones that were more often listed were: lack of interest in sex, not having faith in the future, feeling irritable, not having a clear mind, and not feeling needed and useful.

Physical Symptoms Questionnaire

The women did not score high on this questionnaire, which shows that they suffer mostly from symptoms other than just physical ones.

In all of the women, there was a change in perceiving and feeling their physical symptoms. This was related to the age and general lifestyle of the woman, but in general, most of the symptoms changed from "always felt" to "strongly felt," "strongly felt" to "sometimes felt," or "sometimes felt" to "never felt."

"Always felt" decreased from 7 percent to 4 percent; "strongly felt" from 19 percent to 10 percent; "sometimes felt" from 40 percent to 37 percent; and "never felt" increased from 34 percent to 49 percent.

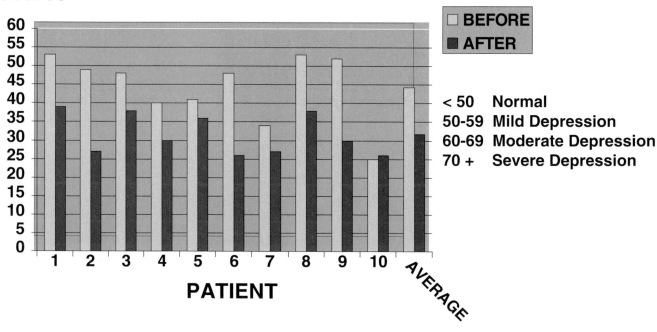

RESULTS OF DEPRESSION TEST

BEFORE
AFTER

< 50   Normal
50-59   Mild Depression
60-69   Moderate Depression
70 +   Severe Depression

Flower Essence Questionnaire

The following is a summary of the answers given by the women when they responded to the questions on the *Flower Essence Society's* Client Background Information form:

Have you used flower essences before? Sometimes; never.

How did you find out about them? Through a therapist; through friends; because they are "alternative remedies."

Describe briefly your general state of health. Sugar in bloodstream; feeling of heart oppression because of anxiety and fear; arthritis; heart infarction ten years before and thrombosis five years before; obesity; an "uncontrolled" menopause; diets; different minor ailments of old age.

Describe briefly your general emotional state. Profound sadness because of mother's death; avoidance of being alone; resentment because of giving more than receiving; depression due to not having done what one wanted; anxiety crisis; depression and low-esteem feeling; perception of being worthless to others; emotional ups and downs.

Describe briefly your general mental state. Feeling of not having succeeded in fulfilling whatever one desired.

Describe briefly your general spiritual state. Feeling of void; looking for definition and depth.

Describe briefly your feelings about work and other vocational interests. Fulfilling work, but little energy and concentration; interest in starting new projects; interest in new challenges; fulfilling job, but tiredness because of not being taken into account; need to express creativity and need to have strength to begin projects.

Describe briefly your feelings in relation to major relationships. Confusing; conflictive; loneliness; feeling of being surrounded by egotism; bad relationships with partner and children.

What other therapies or significant growth experiences have you had? Psychoanalysis, Zen meditation, Gestalt therapy, polarity therapy, body integration therapy, Feldenkreis therapy.

Flower Essences Used

During the study, a general emotional imbalance was reported before menstruation. Even in irregular cycles, the irritation was felt every month. In a previous paper[2], "body memory" was mentioned: the body recalls premenstrual symptoms (PMS) from the start in adolescence until the end of life. These symptoms are fundamental in the psychology of the woman and show her most profound needs. Because this issue was so common, the menopause formula included **Scleranthus** (to address indecision and confusion) and **Walnut** (to move towards a new psychic identity), along with other flower essences chosen to relate to the personality of each individual woman. Each woman's formula was used throughout the whole study. Additional essences for particular problems and feelings were issued when necessary during each session.

This pilot study has shown the effectiveness of flower essence therapy in treating midlife crisis in women.

The problems that arose had to do mainly with issues of indecisiveness and insecurity, depression, libido, menopausal and age-related physical developments, fears, poor sleeping habits, concentration and attention difficulties, problems in relationship with partner, family patterns, resentment, and uncertainty in defining life projects and goals.

The graph on the next page shows the different reasons why the women chose to use flower essences. As the graph shows, almost all the positive items increased in the last evaluation, confirming the state of awareness that flower essence therapy produces, and the fact that it enhances general growth in all spheres of human consciousness.

REASONS FOR TAKING FLOWER ESSENCE REMEDIES

REASONS

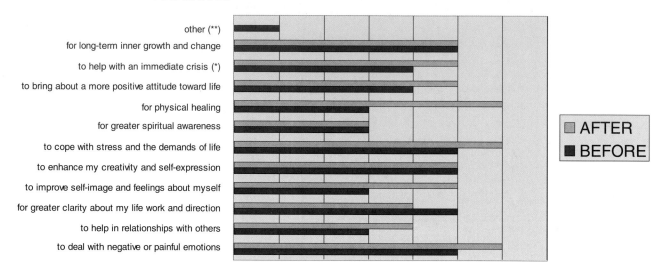

other (**)
for long-term inner growth and change
to help with an immediate crisis (*)
to bring about a more positive attitude toward life
for physical healing
for greater spiritual awareness
to cope with stress and the demands of life
to enhance my creativity and self-expression
to improve self-image and feelings about myself
for greater clarity about my life work and direction
to help in relationships with others
to deal with negative or painful emotions

AFTER
BEFORE

QUANTITATIVE
ANALYSIS

(*) Grief because of mother´s death
Feeling of powerlessness in front of children
Deep void and feeling that life isn´t worth living
Looking for the prime of life
Emotional imbalance and stress
(**) Balance; overcome feelings of frustration; overcome failure

Conclusions

This pilot study has shown the effectiveness of flower essence therapy in treating midlife crisis in women.

It has also shown the importance of the various dimensions of a woman's life, in addition to physical health, that are involved during this period.

Because this group of women was small and all were professionals with a common socio-economic background, the results of this study cannot be applied to all women. Therefore, it will be necessary to conduct wider research that includes a higher population of women from different social and educational backgrounds.

A comparative study of women taking HRT and natural remedies will also be important. Future studies will need to consider the measurement instruments used, and will need to include scales of self-value and life perspective — important issues that became apparent during this pilot study.

End Notes

1 Some of them had both a university degree and professional training.

2 Heyns, Elizabeth, "Emotional Unbalance, Menopause and Flower Essences," paper presented at the IX International Congress of Flower Essence Therapists in Mexico, October, 2002.

Bibliography

Álvarez-Gayou Jurgensen, Juan Luis, *Sexualidad en la pareja,* Manual Moderno, México, 1996.

Bach, Edward, *Los remedios florales. Escritos y conferencias. Las enseñanzas del fundador de la Terapia Floral sobre la esencia de la enfermedad y la salud.* Edaf, Madrid, 1996.

Baker Miller, Jean, *Toward a New Psychology of Women,* Beacon Press, Boston, 1984.

Blome, Götz, *El Nuevo manual de la curación por las Flores de Bach,* Océano, México, 1998.

Espeche, Bárbara and Grecco, Eduardo, *Jung y Flores de Bach. Arcqueotipos y flores,* Ediciones Continente, Buenos Aires, 1993.

Estrada Inda, Lauro, *El ciclo vital de la familia,* Grijalbo, México, 1997.

Grecco, Eduardo, *Sexo, amor y esencias florales,* Ediciones Continente, Argentina, 2001.

Grecco, Eduardo and Bárbara Espeche, *Flores de California: Manual práctico y clínico,* Ediciones Continente, Buenos Aires, 1992.

Grecco, Eduardo, Espeche, Barbara and María A. Valdez, *Flores de California II: Sistemas de esencias pluralistas. Repertorio de síntomas,* Ediciones Continente, Buenos Aires, 1993.

Greer, Germaine, *El cambio. Mujeres, vejez y menopausia,* Anagrama, Barcelona, 1993.

Kaminski, Patricia, *Flowers that Heal. How to Use Flower Essences,* Gill and Macmillan, Dublin, 1998.

Kaminski, Patricia and Katz, Richard, *Flower Essence Repertory: A Comprehensive Guide to North American and English Flower Essences for Emotional and Spiritual Well-Being,* The Flower Essence Society, Nevada City, 1994.

Lara, Luis Fernando, *Diccionario Usual del Español de México* (DUEM), El Colegio de México, México, 1996.

Lara, María Asunción, *¿Es difícil ser mujer? Una guía sobre la depresión,* Instituto Mexicano de Psiquiatría, México, 1997.

Lowenthal, Marjorie and David Chiriboga, "Transition to the Empty Nest: Crisis, Challenge or Relief?", *Archives of General Psychiatry,* 26, January, 1972.

Masters, William H., Johnson, Virginia E. and Kolodry, Robert C., *La sexualidad humana,* Grijalbo, Barcelona, 1995.

McCary, James Leslie, McCary, Stephen, Álvarez-Gayou, Juan Luis, del Río, Carlos José, and Suárez, Luis, *Sexualidad humana de McCary,* Manual Moderno, 1996.

Nolen, Dr. William A., *La crisis del hombre maduro,* Vergara, Buenos Aires, 1985.

Northrup, Christiane, *Women's Bodies, Women's Wisdom: Creating Physical and Emotional Health and Healing,* Bantam Books, NY, 1994.

Northrup, Christiane, *The Wisdom of Menopause. Creating Physical and Emotional Health and Healing During the Change,* Bantam Books, NY, 2001.

Northrup, Christiane, *Women's Bodies, Women's Choices,* JWA Video Audiocassette, 1998.

Robin, Jean Marie, *Contacto y relación en psicoterapia. Reflexiones sobre psicoterapia Gestalt,* Editorial Cuatro Vientos, Santiago de Chile, 1999.

Rodríguez, Segismundo, *Salud en el climaterio y menopausia: Una visión al futuro,* Ediciones Dabar, México, 1997.

Scheffer, Mechthild, *Terapia original de las flores de Bach,* Paidós, Barcelona, 1994.

Sheehy, Gail, *Las crisis de la edad adulta: Cómo superar la angustia de envejecer,* Grijalbo, 1984.

Sheehy, Gail, *Transiciones: Comprender las fases de la madurez en la vida de los hombres,* Urano, Barcelona, 1999.

Souza, Mario and Machorro, *Dinámica y evolución de la vida en pareja,* Manual Moderno, México, 1996.

Willi, Jürg, *La pareja humana: relación y conflicto,* Morata, Madrid, 1993.

Zárate, Arturo and Mac Gregor, Carlos, *Menopausia y cerebro: Aspectos psicosexuales y neurohormonales de la mujer climatérica,* Trillas, México, 1998.

Zung, WW, "A Self-Rating Depression Scale," *Archive of General Psychiatry.* 1965 Jan; 12:63-70.

Silvia: An Illustrative Case of Flower Essences for Menopause

Silvia[1] came asking for help because she said her life was "upside down." She slept poorly and was experiencing PMS (premenstrual syndrome) with great emotional imbalance, including anxiety, fear, and a loss of emotional control.

Silvia is not very tall, and although she is not overweight, she diets constantly, and has always found herself unattractive. She is 41 years old, has been married for six years, and has no children. She is a successful artist with ample work opportunities.

Silvia was born into a high-society Mexican family. Her father was a renowned artist who always encouraged her creativity, but never felt any of her artistic works to be 100 percent perfect.

Her husband is the same age as she. Since their marriage, he has worked very little, so she is the one who supports the household financially. He did not criticize her work — which supported him economically — but criticized her personally. Their sexual life was rather inactive.

Days before menstruating, Silvia felt anxious, irritable, and "in a bad mood." She was also generally depressed, deeply anxious, with nightmares.

Silvia is shown as Patient No. 1 in the Menopause Study. Her anxiety test results show clearly the benefit of using flower essence therapy.

Specific Results

In the physical area: Silvia reduced her anxiety both in number of items and intensity. The most important change was in her ability to sleep well and end her nightmares. I ascribe these changes particularly to the flower essences **Morning Glory** and **White Chestnut**[2].

The most surprising change in the psychological area was the reduction of more than 50 percent in the intensity of symptoms. This was expressed in feeling decreased fear, insecurity, sadness, loss of control of emotions and existential void. **Larch** was first used for her soul condition, followed by

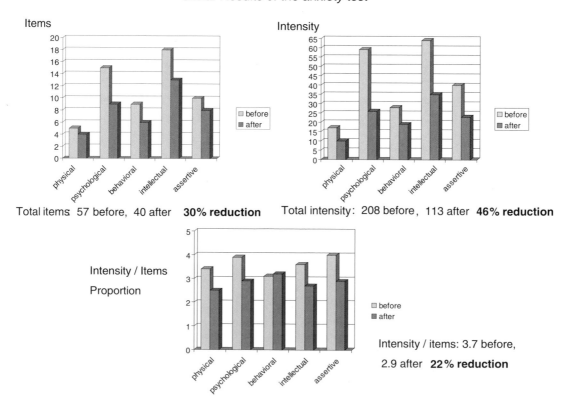

Silvia: Results of the anxiety test

Total items 57 before, 40 after **30% reduction**

Total intensity: 208 before, 113 after **46% reduction**

Intensity / items: 3.7 before, 2.9 after **22% reduction**

Echinacea. This latter essence became one of the most important flower essences used with this patient because it addressed her core spiritual identity, especially her feelings of humiliation and insecurity. **Lavender** and **Chamomile** were also selected for irritability and uneasiness. **Larch** was selected from the beginning for her lack of confidence about her creative work.

At the beginning of treatment, her intellectual area showed the highest level of anxiety. Silvia's anxiety in this area decreased 28 percent in number of items, 45 percent in intensity, and 25 percent in proportion of intensity/items. She showed better memory, although still not 100 percent[3]; overcame her obsessive ideas and worries; and increased her objectivity and positive thinking.

A considerable number of essences where used for issues involving creativity, due to the importance that artistic work plays in Silvia's life. Her first feeling about her creativity was one of complete defeat, a sense of having reached the bottom of the well, the end of the world, and despair. **Scotch Broom** and **Penstemon** were given so that she could continue working, as she had already made commitments and was terrified about being able to complete them. When she had overcome these feelings, she wanted to access her own inspiration, so at that point, **Lotus** and **Iris** were given. Iris also helped her to have a more positive attitude and less critical view toward her work. She then encountered moments of uncertainty and blockage, which she overcame with **Blackberry** and **Peppermint**. At the end of six months, Silvia reported more satisfaction and optimism. She realized the need to change and move in another direction with her creative expression. Therefore, she ended her treatment with **Sagebrush**.

Finally, Silvia's assertive identity improved; she no longer felt insecure when surrounded by people, and actually reported that she grew to like social gatherings because she no longer found it difficult to express her feelings and ideas. While **Scarlet Monkeyflower** was used as part of the treatment in this area, **Echinacea** was the main essence administered.

The first evaluation of depression (53) showed that Silvia was going through a stage of depression due to reactions of anxiety shown on Zung's scale. After six months, the level of depression decreased to normal (39).

Physical menopausal symptoms also decreased in her case. Some symptoms disappeared (16 percent overall). Silvia found 8 percent of symptoms "very little improved," 3 percent "more improved," and symptoms that she described as being "always present" improved 5 percent. Memory, cellulite, softness of skin, quality of sleep, digestive problems, sense of depression, tiredness, anxiety, and despair were reported as improved. Silvia's PMS symptoms also improved: she became aware of what she was feeling, and therefore reduced her anxiety. The length of her PMS also decreased, to only one day of discomfort. Her low libido and vaginal dryness did not improve, although several essences were tried in this area (**Hibiscus, Pomegranate** and **Self-Heal**). Toward the end of the study, she began to feel cramps.

The flower essence Client Evaluation Form showed an increase in her interest for spiritual awareness and personal growth. She decided to go on working with flower essences in the future.

Case follow-up: after another four months of flower essence therapy, Silvia has made more progress. She says that she is redefining herself, and that flower essence therapy has been the most important friend in her journey to do so.

End Notes

1 "Silvia" is not the subject's real name; the rest of the narrative is factual.

2 It is very important to point out that while I will describe specific flower essences related to specific disorders, I want to emphasize that flower essences influence each other mutually, boosting a specific effect or altering an effect when combined. It is also important to point out that essences have different effects when given at a specific time or in a specific sequence in the therapeutic process.

3 Memory problems seem to be one of the general issues that shows up during menopause in most women, including all of my patients.

WomanPause: Understanding the Body-Soul Dynamics of Menopause

By Patricia Kaminski

Scarlet Monkeyflower
Mimulus cardinalis

At age 48, Alice entered into full-blown menopausal symptoms rapidly and with little warning. Alice was a highly successful career woman who married late and who gave birth to her only child at age 44. But rather than enjoying her young daughter, she found herself completely exhausted and full of emotional turmoil. She suffered from debilitating hot flashes and drenching night sweats. In addition, she developed urinary incontinence, making it difficult to get adequate rest at night. After nursing her child, her periods had become scanty and irregular for one year and then ceased altogether. Her medical doctor had prescribed HRT (hormone replacement therapy) for her. However, after 6 months on this therapy, Alice sought an alternative treatment. While on HRT her experience of hot flashes and night sweats subsided, but she had developed many PMS-like symptoms, including bloating, tender breasts, bouts of nausea and weight gain. She still had bladder control problems at night and reported feeling even more tense and moody, and generally exhausted.

As a flower essence counselor, my approach to menopause is unique. While I may recommend herbal and nutritional supplements or work in tandem with other health professionals such as an acupuncturist or nutritionist, I have found that flower essences can play a major role in resolving menopausal transitions by addressing the *soul issues* which women face during this significant life phase. Herbal and nutritional supplements can alleviate the *physical symptoms* which women face in menopause, but it is also vitally important to help each woman understand her own body's expressions as larger messages for change and transformation. When the body is understood from this larger perspective, women do more than adjust to or reverse uncomfortable menopausal symptoms — they develop depth and maturity and move confidently toward menopause as a positive phase of life metamorphosis.

When I first saw Alice, our immediate goal was to wean her from HRT, which was creating havoc in her body. We used a herbal formula specifically indicated for her hormonal profile, which consisted of Black Cohosh (*Cimicifuga racemosa*), Dong Quai (*Angelica sinensis*) and Chasteberry (*Vitex agnus castus*). I also recommended that she add a combination of Evening Primrose, Black Currant and Borage oils to her diet along with an increase of calcium-rich foods such as dark leafy greens.

These herbal and nutritional supplements helped her to cope without synthetic hormones, although her hot flashes and night sweats returned in a less pronounced form.

I initiated flower essence therapy with one single remedy, **Scarlet Monkeyflower** (*Mimulus cardinalis*), to help her address the sensation of hot flashes and night sweats from a deeper level. Scarlet Monkeyflower is a bright red flower with many fiery qualities, yet it grows in a shady environment near flowing streams. It helps to bring deep primal feelings of anger or other forms of "raw fire" into more harmonious or flowing emotional expression. Seen from a larger metaphor of the soul, the hot flashes and night sweats which many women produce in their bodies during menopause are a way in which the alchemy of fire and water need to come to new resolution. With the help of Scarlet Monkeyflower, Alice did not resist her symptoms, but rather moved toward them, and began to experience their deeper impulses for the first time. I had requested that she

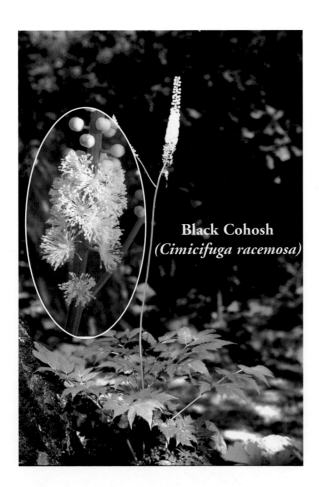

Black Cohosh
(*Cimicifuga racemosa*)

keep a journal about these experiences and she wrote, "I felt a burning wave of energy pass over my body from below, spreading upwards until my neck was red hot and my skin prickled. ... I became fascinated with these waves of energy which periodically washed over me. They went beyond a physical dimension and seemed to connect me with a deep part of myself. ... I began to experience these movements in my body from a different level. I could breathe into and with them, as though they were labor pains. I began to feel I was giving birth to some new part of myself." One evening, when Alice awoke from a night sweat, she also recalled fragments of an intense dream, during which she was expressing deep anger toward her mother. Gradually she uncovered many painful memories and emotions and she wrote, "I feel now as though a flame is burning in me, purifying and illumining me — helping me to see many emotions which I have repressed for a long time. As I raise my young daughter, I am re-visiting parts of my own early relationship with my mother, which were never consciously addressed but only buried. I've always been seen by others as a helper and pleaser — that's what I do in my professional work. But inside, another part of me is ready to explode."

Herbal and nutritional supplements can alleviate the physical symptoms which women face in menopause, but it is also vitally important to help each woman understand her own body's expressions as larger messages for change and transformation.

As Alice assimilated the core message of Scarlet Monkeyflower over a course of about two months, most of the intense symptoms of the hot flashes and night sweats subsided, along with her need for frequent urination. More predominant now were symptoms of deep fatigue, punctuated by brief bouts of nervous hyperactivity. Alice felt, "I need to find a truer source of energy for myself — the old ways just aren't working anymore." At this point, I developed a flower essence master combination for Alice which combined plant remedies from two important families: the lilies and the roses. With their affinity to water and their round bulbs with shallow roots, the lilies have long been associated in herbal and artistic tradition with the cosmic feminine. On the other hand, the rose family plants have deep roots and sharp thorns, and work to transform the will or masculine element within the soul. Seen from an alchemical viewpoint, menopause signals a time when each woman moves from the reproductive and childbearing aspects of the feminine role toward a new expression of her creativity which necessarily incorporates her inner masculine side. Thus, the roses and lilies often work beautifully together to support the new soul alchemy which women need.

The flower essences selected for Alice were **Tiger Lily** (*Lilium humboldtii*), a remedy which helps stabilize the masculine elements within a balanced feminine matrix and **Mariposa Lily** (*Calochortus leichtlinii*), a remedy particularly important for Alice since it address the basic mother archetype of warmth and nurturance. Mariposa Lily is indicated whenever there are issues of relatedness to one's own mother, or doubts or conflicts about one's mothering abilities. Although Alice had many natural mothering abilities which she

used for her professional success, she harbored many internal conflicts which came to the surface in raising her daughter. The final Lily remedy was **Alpine Lily** (*Lilium parvum*), helping Alice to sustain and heal the biological demands of late motherhood, and to also stay present to the actual physical expressions of her body, rather than denying or masking them as she tended to do.

The Rose flower essences for Alice included **California Wild Rose** (*Rosa californica*), a plant essence which brings renewed vitality and enthusiasm by helping instill a new sense of passion or vision for one's life; **Quince** (*Chaenomeles speciosa*), a remedy often recommended for those with a "helper or pleaser" personality, by giving more authentic strength and firmness to one's expressions; and **Blackberry** (*Rubus ursinus*), a remedy which helps to re-vitalize the will forces, especially granting a new sense of life direction and purpose. In addition to taking these flower essences internally, they were also prepared in a base of Self-Heal creme, to which was added several drops of pure rose essential oil; this formula was massaged twice a day into the heart/chest area of her body.

During this time, Alice experienced profound changes both in her body and in her emotions. Over a course of approximately three months, she experienced a renewed sense of energy and purpose.

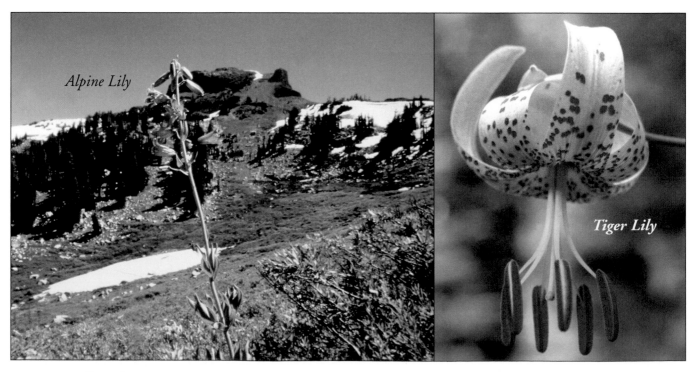

Alpine Lily

Tiger Lily

She no longer reported feelings of utter exhaustion and unexplained fatigue. She made some changes in her career commitments, working less days and being home with her young daughter more. Some tension surfaced in her relationship with her husband, as she expressed her needs rather than stifling her resentments. However, she viewed the relationship as more honest, authentic and positively dynamic than it had previously been. She began to develop new plans for her career, including consulting work from her home, which proved to be more lucrative and allowed her more time with her family. She also enrolled in an art course which helped her to find expression for new parts of herself. This was something she had always wanted to make time for, but felt previously that she would be "selfish" to do so. Most surprising of all, her menstrual period returned for approximately two more years. She reported, "I used to feel annoyed by my period and couldn't wait for it to be over. Then I mourned the fact that it had been lost to me so suddenly. Now I treasure every moment of this special time with my body; I feel graced to have a second chance to complete this part of my life cycle and I want to be present for every minute of it." About a year after using these flower essences, Alice reported feeling like an entirely different person. She gave this insight, "I don't want to see menopause as 'fixing' my biological clock. I have never felt more excited about my future. I *want* to move forward. I feel I am a completely different person than I was two years ago. I have gone through a dark tunnel and come out the other side."

There are many other important flower essences which can be used for helping women through the transition of menopause. Each woman is an individual and has unique life issues which she alone must encounter and transform. These issues come to expression in the body but they are far larger than the body. I have come to call this special time **WomanPause**, for it is truly a time when each woman must be helped to reflect upon her life values, to reclaim her physical body, and to develop a new sense of dignity, maturity and wisdom about who she is as a soul-spiritual being.

Leading Flower Essences for Menopause

Flower essences provide outstanding support for the mental and emotional issues which women encounter during the menopausal years. They are used very successfully with other health modalities such as chiropractic, acupuncture, nutrition and herbalism, and help to bring a deeper soul dimension of healing to each woman's experience of menopause.

Alpine Lily *Lilium parvum* — Helps women to integrate the bodily experience of menopause; to move through physical sensations of pain or discomfort toward a deeper sense of the feminine.

Angelica *Angelica archangelica* — The herbal Angelica (called Dong Quai) is a classic women's remedy. However, this form of Angelica brings an even deeper sense of expansiveness and spiritual relatedness. It helps to relieve the sense of compression or diminishment many women experience during menopause. Instead, one can re-discover a larger sense of self and soul purpose.

Black Cohosh *Cimicifuga racemosa* — This herb is well known for its estrogen-balancing qualities, but when used as a flower essence, it works more energetically to open up blocked energy in the entire pelvic region. It is especially important for women who feel intense feelings of anger, rage or violence during the menopausal transition. It is also helpful for painful and debilitating menstrual cycles.

California Wild Rose *Rosa californica* — Helps women who feel drained or exhausted during menopause, or who tend to look back to a past life phase rather than forward to their future.

Fairy Lantern *Calochortus albus* — For women who resist the developmental phase of menopause, especially a psychological need to remain young in an inappropriate way. For a deep fear of aging, or of being seen as "mature."

Hibiscus *Hibiscus rosa-sinensis* — For physical or emotional "dryness," reduced sexual response or sensation. For helping to re-define one's sense of sexuality and integrating soul warmth with physical desire.

Lady's Mantle *Alchemilla vulgaris* — An excellent all purpose flower essence during menopause, helping women to find a larger, positive feminine identity, especially an ability to sense one's physical body as being nurtured by the larger physical.

Mariposa Lily *Calochortus leichtlinii* — For completing the mothering phase of life or for the empty-nest syndrome. Also, for helping to transform deep-seated beliefs or superstitions about menopause internalized from one's mother/grandmother.

Pomegranate *Punica granatum* — A major flower essence for menopause, helping women redirect the psychic and physical forces of procreativity and reproduction to *soul creativity*. An important essence for experiencing menopause as a positive and natural outcome of the feminine identity.

Quince *Chaenomeles speciosa* — Helping women to combine the softer, more feminine and yielding aspects of their identity with emergent feelings of strength and power associated with the inner masculine of each woman's soul.

Sage *Salvia officinalis* — Helps to refine the over-abundance of watery emotions into calmer, more objective feelings. Instills the ability to reflect on life experience and see the movements of one's life from a larger perspective. One of the flower essences which can be very helpful for "water" problems during menopause such as increased sweating and frequent urination.

Sagebrush *Artemisia tridentata* — Addresses the emptiness many women feel during menopause, as a positive experience. Helps to bring a sense of inner stillness, or "pause." Also a deeply cleansing remedy to release accumulated physical and psychic toxins which must be cleared before a new life phase can begin.

Scarlet Monkeyflower *Mimulus cardinalis* — Very helpful flower essence for helping to see hot flashes and other fire manifestations during menopause at a deeper emotional level. This flower essence especially addresses repressed emotional material, such as anger, which may be blocking the vitality and physical energy.

Tiger Lily *Lilium humboldtii* — To help integrate and balance many energetic fluctuations during menopause, especially helping the masculine forces to remain integrated with the deep feminine.

Walnut *Juglans regia* — An excellent stabilizing remedy during menopause, helping women to break old links or dysfunctional identities and move forward with a renewed sense of soul purpose and identity.

Yarrow *Achillea millefolium* — For women who become over-sensitive during menopause and too emotionally expanded. Also, for many physical symptoms such as prolonged menstrual bleeding or "flooding."

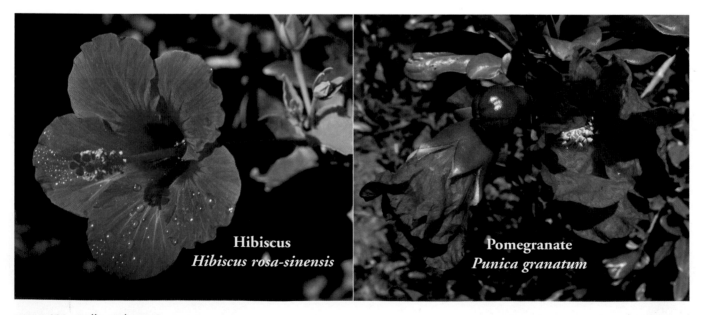

Hibiscus
Hibiscus rosa-sinensis

Pomegranate
Punica granatum

Fertility and the Feminine Soul

Flower essences help a young woman become pregnant

a case report from Mitose Komura

You should not treat the body without the soul.

Plato's Dialogues

*Editor's Note: The following is a summary of a fully documented case submitted to the **FES Certification Program** by Mitose Komura. This case shows the remarkable transformation within the body and soul of a 27-year old Japanese woman. Diagnosed with severe endometriosis, Hanako was challenged with depression, physical pain and a troubled feminine identity. This case is significant not only for showing how Hanako resolves her soul and bodily pain, but also how the flower essences work in a positive, complimentary manner along with standard medical intervention. Therapeutic sketches from the client provide dramatic examples of the soul's transformative steps toward recovery.*

Client Background — "I Want to Accept Being a Woman and Mother"

Hanako sought flower essence therapy because she realized she was very unhappy in her identity as a woman. Hanako looked much younger than her biological age of 27, with her slender, delicate and child-like features. Although a graduate of a Japanese university and employed by a legal firm, Hanako was unhappy in her work. She believed that many women in her country were treated with "social unfairness." She was born with a twin brother and felt the difference in their social status, despite being his equal. Hanako was estranged from her mother, who neglected her as a child in favor of her twin brother. She grew up feeling that she did not want to be like her mother.

Hanako was happily married and wanted to have a child but attempts to do so had not been successful. She suffered from endometriosis, with menstrual pain so debilitating she had to miss work each month. She hoped that the flower essences could resolve her medical condition, help her conceive a child, and achieve a more positive understanding of her identity as a woman. She wrote on her client intake form, "I want to accept being a woman and a mother."

Hanako's drawings demonstrate how therapeutic art can express the soul's healing journey. Beginning with a fall into a dark abyss, she reveals isolation and hopelessness. As she heals, she opens a door into a new, vibrant, life-affirming world.

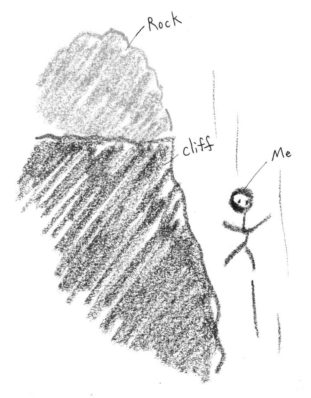

① "Falling off a cliff"
··· Around when I started taking the essence.
(November, 1998 ~)

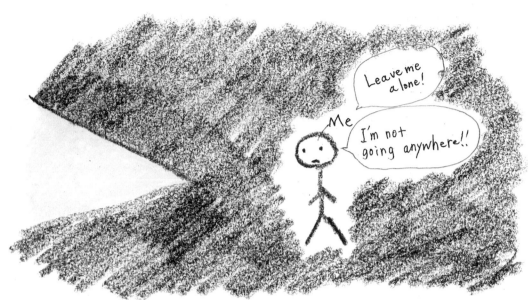

② "A Light closing in around me day by day." (Feb.,1999 ~ May, 1999)
··· I didn't want to see anyone and cut as many thinkable contacts as possible.
It lasted a couple months until I finally got tired of it and accepted the fact that
I would have an operation.

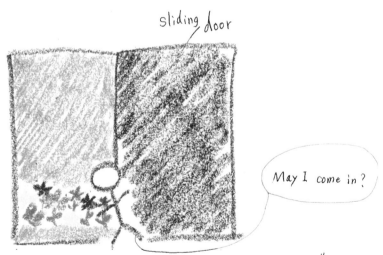

③ "Peeping into a new world full of flowers, green and insects."
··· After hospitalization (May 20, 1999 ~). They took out my left ovary,
but now I'm free of the pain I used to feel, and each day brings me
happiness and teaches me how beautiful the world is.

Major Flower Essences in Hanako's Case

Mariposa Lily — This essence was foundational for Hanako. It helped her to acknowledge the relationship with her mother, healing the wounds she felt. This flower guided her to find the true soul archetype of what it means to be a mother. It cleansed the distortion of the archetype she felt in childhood, clearing her soul's path to motherhood.

Alpine Lily — This essence addressed the alienation Hanako felt for her female identity. Her bodily identity and soul identity were in great stress and conflict, not flowing together. This discord manifested in her severe endometriosis.

Angelica — Angelica helped Hanako realize a higher spiritual identity, one that could awaken her to new directions and new values in her life. Angelica also provided a sense of protection and support during her time of suffering and despair as she healed herself and re-patterned her life.

Black-Eyed Susan — This essence was used to address Hanako's depression and feelings of darkness as the symptoms of endometriosis worsened. The metaphor of congestion in Hanako's womb was reflected in her soul and is revealed in the drawings accompanying this article. Hanako began to "see" the darkness in her soul, and she brought it into a meeting with light.

Fawn Lily — Hanako came more fully into her body and social relationships through the use of the Fawn Lily. This Lily represents Hanako's constitutional type and worked in a strong archetypal way in the therapy. Her slender and delicate body gives the impression of a soul type who remains aloof. She stays in the upper chakras of her feminine identity. Further, because of her troubling relationship with her mother and her larger cultural identity, she did not come fully into her body or into social relationships. Hanako writes, "I am the type of person who refuses others' help in a bad situation."

Gentian — Hanako experienced core levels of depression and discouragement. Gentian addressed those feelings, especially when Hanako found her endometriosis was not immediately resolved.

Evening Primrose — This essence healed the core wound in Hanako's physical reproductive system. This is the wound that originated from her psychic experience in the womb of her mother. Her alienation continued throughout childhood with feelings that her mother rejected her and preferred her male twin brother. Hanako wanted to be a mother yet she feared becoming like her own mother.

Mugwort — Mugwort brought warmth and healing forces to Hanako's reproductive system, especially the lunar element that is associated with the menstrual cycle. The Mugwort was also used to integrate the psychic or lunar forces of Hanako's soul with her physical reality. During the course of treatment, Hanako's psychic awareness greatly increased. She experienced dream recall and other soul images that she felt inspired to sketch.

Pomegranate — Hanako's ambivalence about her career and her desires for motherhood — particularly as these issues played into her feminine reproductive system — were resolved with the help of Pomegranate essence.

Love-Lies-Bleeding — For the intense pain and bleeding symptoms Hanako experienced as a result of endometriosis, the Love-Lies-Bleeding was administered. This also helped the psychic effects of this pain that created feelings of isolation.

Red Clover — Red Clover helped Hanako recognize the psychic blood ties in her family system. She was able to recognize how this psychic distress affected her own bleeding abnormalities. Red Clover gave Hanako's soul new containment and individuality, and it was instrumental in rebuilding her blood forces after surgery.

Self-Heal — To connect Hanako with her own healing forces, the Self-Heal essence was used. This flower essence was very important in the remarkable recovery Hanako made after her surgery. Her healing was very speedy and the doctors were astounded to see how quickly she conceived a child. The qualities of Self-Heal are also evident in her third drawing that shows how she opened her soul to the forces of Nature and life renewal.

A Diagnosis of Endometriosis and Fibroid Tumors

The first strategy focused on whether the flower essences could help reverse Hanako's physical condition of severe endometriosis while acknowledging that her condition was already very extreme. One-and-a-half months after beginning flower essence therapy, Hanako's doctor diagnosed her medical condition as advanced endometriosis. A later examination revealed fibroid tumors. The doctor recommended immediate surgery.

The therapeutic strategy was then changed to help Hanako accept the operation and to examine the deeper karma that had led to her condition. Without a healing from within her feminine soul, her body might be changed on the outside, but the patterns that had created dysfunction would continue to work in other ways in her life destiny.

During this time, Hanako began to identify many toxic emotions and experiences that contributed to her current identity. She saw how dramatically the feelings of her soul were affecting her body. For example, when she spoke with her mother on the telephone, her pain became much worse. She had not seen this impact as clearly before she began flower essence therapy.

Dealing with Depression: "Leave Me Alone"

Prior to her surgery, Hanako experienced a period of intensified feelings. This interval was very important from an alchemical point of view, helping her to consciously face the darkness and despair she felt. Hanako feared the operation and wondered whether she would lose her reproductive capacity entirely. It appeared that her condition was getting worse, yet this was actually a beneficial time for her. It helped her through powerful feelings of depression, bringing her to another level of consciousness. As her drawings show, she felt as if she were plunging into a place of darkness (drawing #1), a wall of isolation was building around her, and she was losing hope in the future (drawing #2). These feelings had long been festering in her soul and now they were brought from the hidden depths and made more visible to her. The **Loves-Lies-Bleeding, Gentian** and **Black-Eyed Susan** flower essences were especially important at this time.

Fawn Lily grows in the high mountain meadows as winter's snows melt into summer's streams. It was Hanako's archetypal remedy to help her come more fully into her body and social relationships.

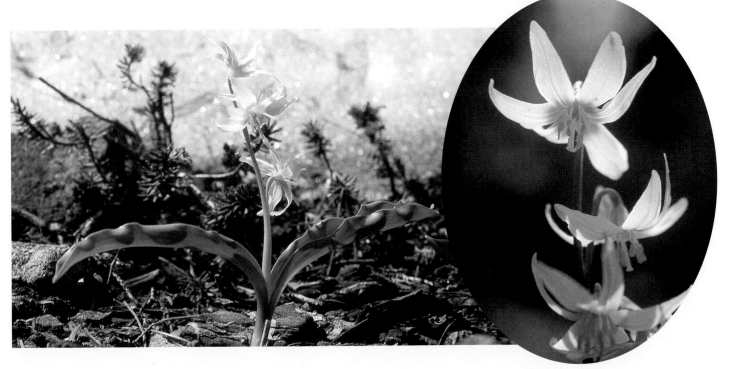

Transformation: "Each Day Teaches Me How Beautiful the World Is"

Hanako went ahead with the operation. This occurred toward the end of the third month of her therapy with flower essences. She had already worked through many of her feelings and had accepted the operation as her best chance for physical recovery. During the operation, her swollen left ovary was removed. Despite the severity of the operation, she made a remarkable recovery. She began to notice green plants and trees and reported that her heart felt open to the beauty of life. She could feel her body being healed very rapidly. Hanako felt renewed hope for her life.

Hanako Conceives a Daughter

Only six months after her surgery, Hanako became pregnant. The doctor was astonished to hear this, calling it "unbelievable." It is very rare for the reproductive system to heal and regenerate itself so rapidly after a major operation. Because Hanako had only one remaining ovary, it meant there were limited opportunities for fertilization in the short six-month time span following her operation.

Hanako had continued her flower essence therapy during those six months along with related modalities such as drawing, affirmations and color therapy. Her soul felt reborn and continued to grow in radiance with a positive outlook. This soul condition opened the channels for her to conceive very rapidly.

Hanako is now the very happy mother of a daughter. She feels that she has resolved many major emotions and has healed many issues in her family system.

Mitose Komura is the director of the *Association for Flower Essence Education* in Japan *(www.afeej.org)*. She teaches many practitioners and is building the foundation for in-depth flower essence therapy in her country. Mitose Komura received her certification from FES and is now overseeing the certification of many Japanese students writing in their native language. In commenting about Hanako's case, Komura says: "It was a precious experience as well as a big challenge for me. I saw the role of flower essences in helping Hanako increase her soul awareness and open her heart. I learned to respect each individual's own way of healing."

Mitose Komura lives in Setagaya-ku, Tokyo and can be reached via e-mail at mail@afeej.org.

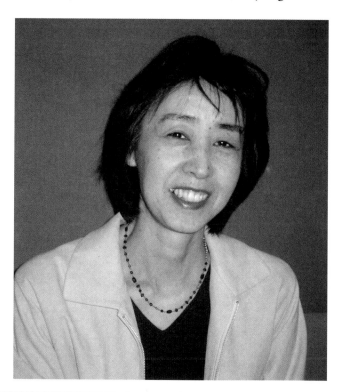

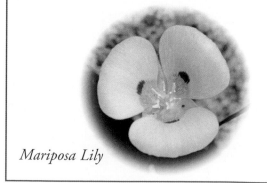

Mariposa Lily

From the heart of the earth we come
The kind Mother of Life and of All
And if you think She is not wise
You should know that flowers are her songs.

Native American Song

Leading Flower Essences for Conception and Pregnancy

by Patricia Kaminski

Alpine Lily *Lilium parvum*

Integrates female bodily identity with feminine spiritual ideals; helps reproductive organs experience conception and pregnancy as positive states; especially beneficial for women challenged by the intense physical experience of pregnancy or weight gain.

Angelica *Angelica archangelica*

Generally beneficial remedy in early stages of pregnancy if prone to miscarriage. Creates spiritual link with incoming child and provides protection and spiritual centering.

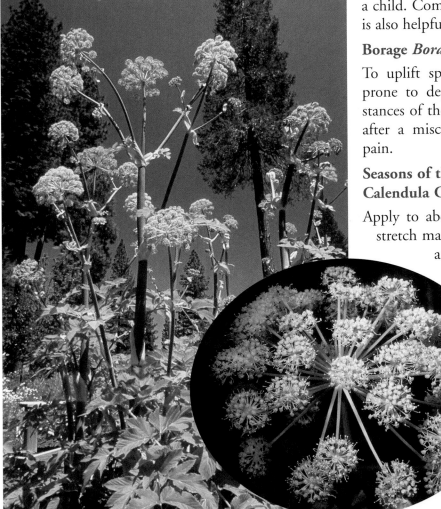

Angelica

Seasons of the Soul Herbal Flower Oil — Benediction Oil

Use anytime throughout pregnancy in full body massage or baths to create a feeling of sacredness and centeredness in the pregnancy. Benediction Oil is especially indicated to open the heart, and feel bonding with the incoming child. Use in full body massage in the weeks prior to pregnancy as preparation for birth.

Bleeding Heart *Dicentra formosa*

Clears the reproductive organs of grief or related emotions from the past that may prevent conception or carrying the child to term. Bleeding Heart is especially indicated for women who have suffered prior miscarriages, abortions, or the death of a child. Combined with **Gentian**, Bleeding Heart is also helpful for post-partum depression.

Borage *Borago officinalis*

To uplift spirits during pregnancy, especially if prone to depression, or if surrounding circumstances of the pregnancy are challenging; for grief after a miscarriage or abortion to soothe heart pain.

Seasons of the Soul Herbal Flower Oil — Calendula Caress

Apply to abdomen during pregnancy to prevent stretch marks, and to breasts to make them soft and supple. Put several tablespoons in warm water bath at night to feel calm, serene and harmonious throughout the pregnancy. Additional drops of **Mariposa Lily, Star Tulip** and **Cerato** can be added to the bath water. Use after pregnancy to restore the skin and heal stretch marks.

California Wild Rose *Rosa californica*

Increases the ability to anchor a new life on Earth; for difficult pregnancies or births; to help the incarnating soul feel the call of love and human warmth on earth. Apply topically to the heart during pregnancy and to the heart and fontanel of newborn child. Topical applications of California Wild Rose and **Shooting Star** on the fontanel are especially important for children who are delivered via cesarean method.

Calla Lily *Zantedeschia aethiopica*

For mixed messages about sexual identity; a strong personal preference for either a male or female child due to cultural bias or prejudice, causing confusion or anxiety for the incarnating soul while *in utero*.

Centaury *Centaurium erythraea*

Overwork and exhaustion during pregnancy, due to an inability to say "no;" meeting others' demands and expectations rather than attending to the true needs of the pregnancy.

Cerato *Ceratostigma willmottiana*

Developing trust in one's inner knowing; relying on the strength of one's sense of choice regarding pre-natal and natal care; learning to make the right health-care and personal care choices by trusting one's innate wisdom. Combines well with **Self-Heal** essence.

Chamomile *Matricaria recutita*

Use Chamomile when prone to crying or other emotional upset during pregnancy to center and balance the emotions. Also helpful for nausea or for leg cramps. Apply topically in **Self-Heal Creme** or take internally.

Chocolate Lily *Fritillaria biflora*

Can be a very beneficial remedy for cleansing reproductive organs and lowering metabolism, particularly congestive conditions such as endometriosis, cysts or intestinal adhesions. This essence is especially related to first and second chakra blockage that may prevent conception or otherwise undermine reproductive health.

Cherry Plum *Prunus cerasifera*

For extremely stressful pregnancy or labor, when irrational states of consciousness erode inner ability to stay with the process of labor; when one feels "I can't take any more."

Corn *Zea mays*

For developing the archetype of the "Earth Mother"; for women who lack strength and grounding during pregnancy; for feet that are tired and sore during later stages of pregnancy, or when feeling too "heavy." Apply topically to the feet.

Easter Lily *Lilium longiflorum*

For cleansing of sexual organs, especially when conception is blocked due to prior sexual trauma or behavior. To help build a healthy bridge from sexuality to conception.

Elm *Ulmus procera*

When over-anxious or over-striving for perfection in parenthood, feeling motherhood as a burden or duty rather than a joy.

Evening Primrose *Oenothera hookeri*

For extreme emotional toxicity during pregnancy, including unconscious or conscious destructive intent to fetus by mother or others. For mothers who may have been adopted or abused in early childhood and who unconsciously transfer emotional fear or rejection to incarnating child.

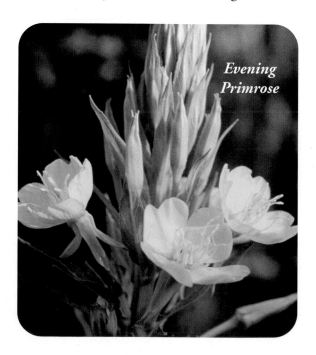

Evening Primrose

Fairy Lantern *Calochortus albus*

For young mothers who are challenged by the adult responsibilities of motherhood. To facilitate the flow of breast milk, especially in young mothers; take internally and apply topically. This remedy combines well with **Mariposa Lily,** a close botanical plant ally.

Five-Flower Formula (also known as Rescue Remedy) — Cherry Plum, Clematis, Impatiens, Rock Rose, Star of Bethlehem

General all-purpose formula for all states of emergency or stress during pregnancy. Extremely beneficial during labor for the mother and attendants to stay calm and centered. Helpful for challenging, stressful or atypical birth situations such as premature birth or delivery via cesarean section. Fosters calm and reduces stress.

Forget-Me-Not *Myosotis sylvatica*

To facilitate conscious conception, especially the awareness of one's karmic connections with the incarnating being.

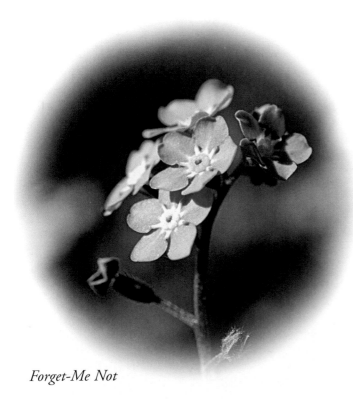

Forget-Me Not

Gentian *Gentiana amarella*

For setbacks during pregnancy or difficulty conceiving. For any state of despondency, including post-partum depression.

Indian Paintbrush *Castilleja miniata*

For low vitality during pregnancy, and for recuperation after pregnancy. Especially indicated if anemic during pregnancy or if significant blood loss occurs during labor.

Joshua Tree *Yucca brevifolia*

To clear genetic and psychic material in the soul of the mother (and father) that arises from the family of origin, culture, religion or community that may challenge or trouble the incarnation of the child (i.e., alcoholism, a marriage of mixed race or religion, etc.)

Lady's Mantle *Alchemilla vulgaris*

Has a generally beneficial role for all reproductive health issues in women. During pregnancy, it helps the larger mothering forces from Nature flow into the blood and nourish the heart and womb. Also facilitates a magnetic, receptive life force conducive to conception.

Lavender *Lavandula officinalis*

For use when the mother is too high-strung or nervous during pregnancy. Effective when used with **Chamomile**. Combined with **Five-Flower Formula**, serves to calm and relax during labor. Apply topically to the temples and forehead.

Manzanita *Arctostaphylos viscida*

Acceptance of physical body during pregnancy; to offset feeling of ugliness or awkwardness in the body; for aversion to food or other eating disorders during pregnancy.

Mariposa Lily *Calochortus leichtlinii*

The single-most important essence for all stages of pregnancy, including conception, delivery and motherhood. Helps build a strong positive sense of mothering identity and bonding with the incoming child. Imparts confidence about one's ability to be a mother and builds rapport between mother and child. *Extremely beneficial and powerful essence combined with others or taken alone.*

Mugwort *Artemisia douglasiana* and Seasons of the Soul Herbal Flower Oil — Mugwort Moon Magic

Recommended only for final stage of pregnancy and during birth. Helps the child drop into position and prepare for birth. Use during labor to promote birthing and delivery of afterbirth. Apply topically to breasts to promote healthy flow of milk. Take flower essence internally and use external applications of Mugwort Moon Magic.

Olive *Olea europaea*

For profound fatigue from missed sleep during pregnancy or exhaustion from long labor.

Penstemon *Penstemon davidsonii*

Gives strength to persevere during challenging and difficult pregnancies, especially when there is stress, challenge, or accompanying physical handicaps or hardships.

Pink Yarrow *Achillea millefolium* var. *rubra*

For extreme over-sensitivity or absorption of others' emotions; emotional vulnerability to influences in the home or workplace when pregnant. Combine with **Angelica** and **Yarrow Environmental Solution** if work or other duties create excessive external demands.

Pomegranate *Punica granatum*

To help direct creative forces during conception and pregnancy, especially when there are conflicts about motherhood, career, or other identities. An important essence for women who need to make a conscious choice about life-destiny issues and mothering.

Quince *Chaenomeles speciosa*

For women who must balance strength and nurturing during pregnancy, such as competence and strength in career duties and receptivity and nurturing in personal life.

Red Chestnut *Aesculus carnea*

For anxiety and concern about pregnancy and the new child; anxious states of mind not directed toward the self, but toward others.

Red Clover *Trifolium pratense*

For states of hysteria or panic during pregnancy, especially if they are connected to family emergencies, "trauma-drama" in the family system, or other "group soul" connection for the pregnant woman. Can be used alone or combined with **Five-Flower Formula** or **Pink Yarrow**, depending on the circumstance. An excellent remedy for cleansing both psychic and physical properties in the blood and "family blood ties" prior to conception. It combines well with **Joshua Tree** for these purposes.

Scarlet Fritillary *Fritillaria recurva*

Helpful for integrating an element of vitality and strength in pregnancy, childbirth and lactation. Especially indicated if anemic, physically weak, exhausted, or poor lactation occurs. Very beneficial when combined with **Indian Paintbrush** for prolonged labor or cesarean birth, especially for loss of blood. Brings vital "red" forces to the mothering experience.

Self-Heal *Prunella vulgaris* and Self-Heal Creme

For any healing challenges or toxic states during pregnancy; to help the body cope with colds, flu, or any other illnesses during pregnancy. Prevents the need for invasive drugs or other harsh medical treatments. Use Self-Heal Creme for any skin afflictions during pregnancy. The creme also serves as a conduit for topical applications of the other flower essences.

Shooting Star *Dodecatheon hendersonii*

To prevent miscarriage at any stage of pregnancy; for trauma during labor or cesarean birth. Especially indicated when the incarnating soul of the child appears conflicted about coming to earth and being in a physical body.

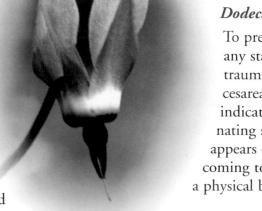

Shooting Star

Star Tulip *Calochortus tolmiei*

Highly beneficial essence during all stages of pregnancy, labor and new motherhood. Helps develop telepathic communication with child, and facilitates inner sense of timing and harmony for each stage of pregnancy and labor. This essence combines very effectively with **Mariposa Lily.**

Tiger Lily *Lilium humboldtii*

To assist in conception and successful pregnancy in older women. To build greater feminine forces in both the body and soul, especially if there is a tendency toward an overly masculine identity.

Walnut *Juglans regia*

Assists in each trimester of development during pregnancy. Especially indicated during labor to help the child and mother "break links" as the child separates from its home in the womb and descends through the birth canal.

White Chestnut *Aesculus hippocastanum*

For insomnia, excessive worry and other obsessive mental states during pregnancy, especially when these thoughts are directed toward the self, rather than others.

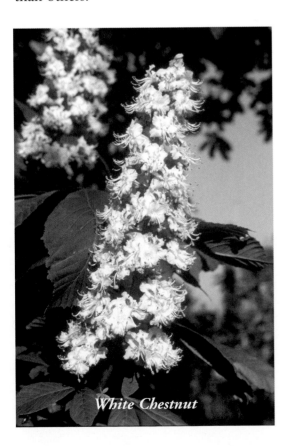

White Chestnut

Yarrow *Achillea millefolium*

For psychic and physical vulnerability during pregnancy; for spotting or bleeding during pregnancy, premature labor, or heavy bleeding during labor. **Pink Yarrow** may also be indicated.

Yarrow Environmental Solution (Yarrow, Pink Yarrow, Golden Yarrow, Arnica, Echinacea)

When exposed to environmental stresses during pregnancy, including radiation or any form of toxicity. Use frequently when traveling, especially when flying. Take internally and apply topically to the abdomen.

Pregnancy Balm

A general all-purpose formula that can be used throughout all stages of pregnancy. The Pregnancy Balm provides positive support and nurturing, and helps the mother stay in touch with her child and her own wisdom throughout the pregnancy. Use when there are no specific indications, troubling emotions or other challenges. Consists of **Mariposa Lily, Star Tulip, Lady's Mantle** and **Cerato.** Pregnancy Balm can be formulated as a regular dosage bottle. Stock drops can also be added to a misting bottle and sprayed over the entire body.

Pregnancy Balm Cream

10 stock drops of any of the above flower essences can be added to **Self-Heal Creme,** along with two drops of Rose Attar pure essential oil, and gently massaged on a daily basis over the womb area.

> The medical school of the future will ... concentrate its efforts upon bringing about the harmony between body, mind and soul, which results in the relief and cure of disease.
>
> Dr. Edward Bach, Heal Thyself

Soul On Fire:

Healing Tobacco Addiction with Flower Essence Therapy

By Patricia Kaminski

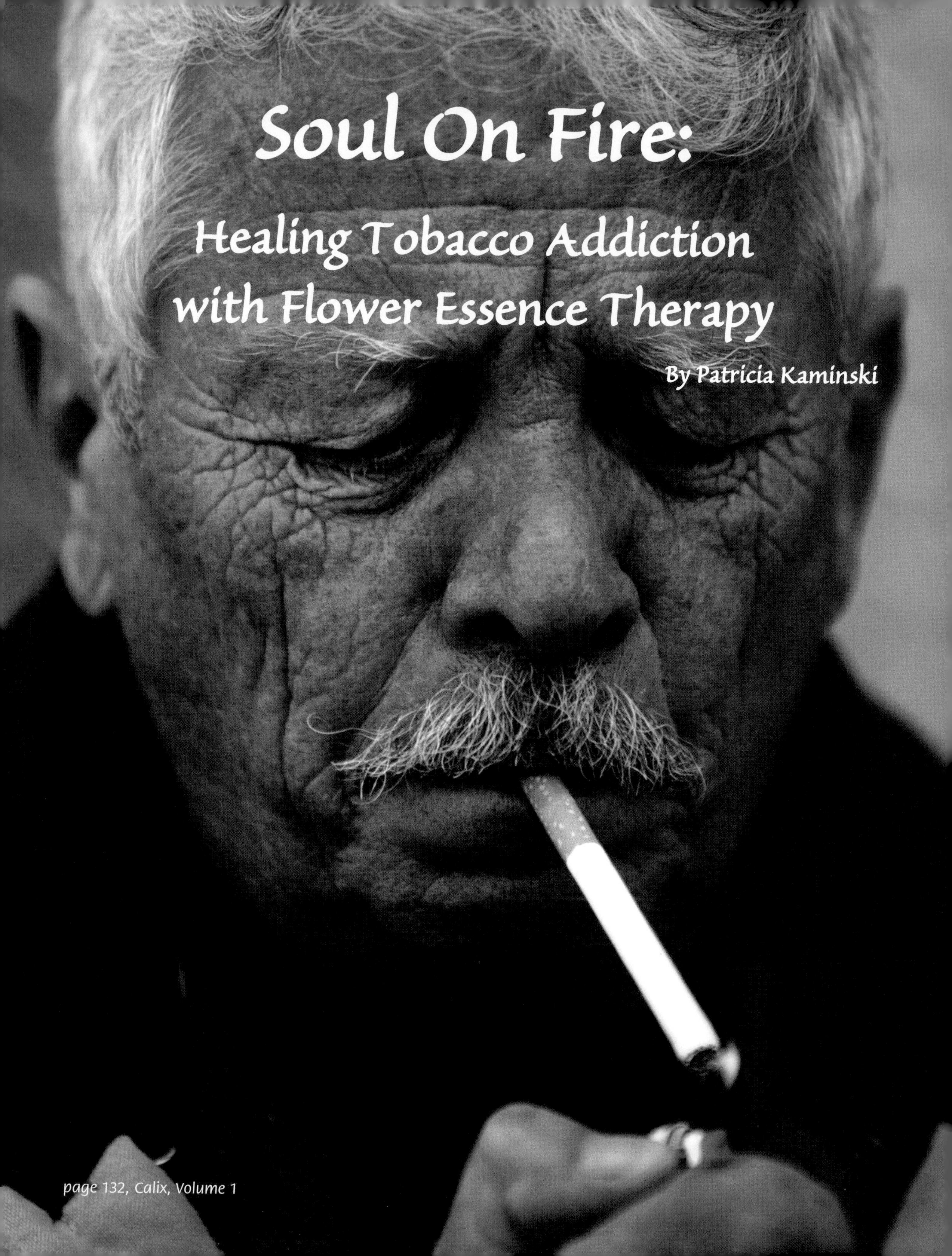

Seeing Inside: The Soul as Bridge to the Body

If the vital organs damaged by nicotine inhalation were on the *outside of the human body*, it is likely that few people would smoke very long. It would take only a short while to see the visible damage of modern tobacco products (containing over 4,000 different chemicals[1]) that congest the heart and lungs, deprive oxygen to the brain, disturb the circulatory system, and cause premature aging through numerous adverse changes in the metabolism and skin tissue.

Perhaps there is a good reason why we do not have instant visible access to the interior reality of the human body. The ability to sense the needs of the physical body depends not merely on physical eyes, but upon soul perception. For this reason, medical facts and technology alone seldom have the moral power to facilitate change. If addiction to nicotine (or any other substance) arises due to a lack of consciousness about our bodies, it is only truly healed when the soul develops a stronger relationship to its bodily identity.

If addiction to nicotine (or any other substance) arises due to a lack of consciousness about our bodies, it is only truly healed when the soul develops a stronger relationship to its bodily identity.

Flower essence therapy can play a significant role in resolving tobacco addiction by helping the individual identify positive qualities that can transform such craving. The unique aim of flower essence therapy is not simply the modification of a "bad" outer behavior, but a healing approach that finds the good within the soul, so that the individual develops greater self-mastery and consciousness. For over two decades, the *Flower Essence Society* has compiled case research from practitioners who are helping clients overcome tobacco addiction. This article covers some of the main highlights of this research.

Tobacco Addiction: Four Fundamental Flowers

One or more of the following four flower essences are foundational in nearly all cases of nicotine addiction. They can be used together or separately as needed. In addition to standard internal dosages, they can be used in creams and baths or saunas, as outlined in the "detox" segment of this article.

Nicotiana — Made from the Native American flowering tobacco (*Nicotiana alata*), this flower essence helps the soul encounter the true spiritual archetype that is at the heart of nicotine craving: the need to bring fire forces to the will, grounded in the calm strength of the body in alignment with the earth. Nicotiana flower essence should be used for all stages of tobacco recovery, and may be indicated for a sustained period of time for heavily addicted users. (Please see plant profile on page 146.)

Yerba Santa — This classic Native American wildflower has a remarkable cleansing effect on the heart and lung region. It clears both physical and emotional congestion, particularly addressing grief, loss, vulnerability and other troubling emotions stored in the chest, lungs and heart. These hidden feelings may be traced back to childhood or other traumatic or karmic life events. They create the emotional "receptor" site that typically serves as a precursor to tobacco addiction. (Please see plant profile on page 148.)

Morning Glory — The natural metabolic rhythms of the body are disrupted through nicotine addiction. Tobacco has an accelerative effect that "jump starts" the heart and circulatory system. Nicotine's powerful hold derives from this false energy state, and the user becomes increasingly dependent upon it for a sense of well-being. Morning Glory helps re-establish natural rhythms of sleeping, eating and working, based on the body's true life energy. Initial use of Morning Glory may result in feelings of fatigue, insomnia, or decreased/increased hunger until the natural balance of the metabolism is re-established.

Borage — An excellent balm for the heart, Borage addresses many aspects of manifest or covert depression associated with nicotine addiction. The toxic effects of such depression are stored in the heart organ and in the energetic pathways associated with the heart chakra. Because the heart rate is accelerated, the acute "heaviness" of the heart is momentarily lifted when smoking, thus creating a desperate cycle of addiction to ease the pain felt in the heart.

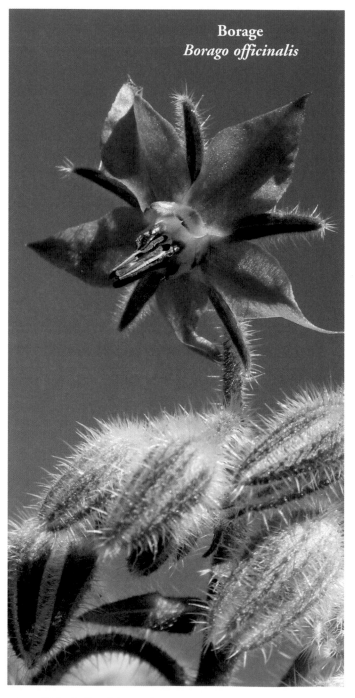

Borage
Borago officinalis

The Nicotine Nexus: Body-Mind Beliefs

Tobacco has been called "the most underestimated drug in the world[2]." Those who have been cross-addicted to other substances like alcohol and heroin, report that tobacco is often a far more difficult habit to break. Many users are caught in a cycle of shame or despair, due to many failed attempts to quit, while others are in strong patterns of denial about the deleterious effects of nicotine. Prior to achieving smoking cessation, it is often necessary to explore core attitudes or beliefs that may be undermining successful termination. The following flower essences should be considered during this process:

Manzanita — A very effective remedy for those individuals who are disconnected from or abusive to their bodies. They typically see the body as "lower," "inessential," "ugly," "handicapped"— or simply not worthy of respect or nourishment. Therefore, it does not "matter" whether the body is being harmed with drugs. Manzanita combines well with Self-Heal to help such individuals come to a spiritual appreciation of the worth of their lives and their bodies.

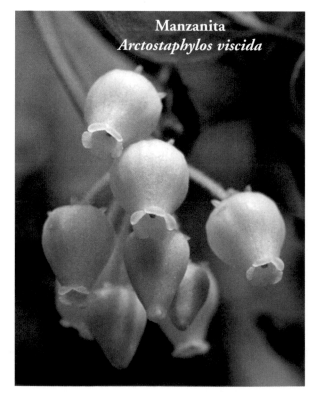

Manzanita
Arctostaphylos viscida

Self-Heal — Stimulates the motivation to be well, to learn to listen to and respect the body's need for health and nourishment. Many who are in denial about the harmful effects of nicotine report becoming acutely conscious of the inner reality of their body and its need for healing. Others find Self-Heal necessary for motivation and inner commitment to the healing process involved in addiction recovery.

Rock Water — Indicated along with Nicotiana for those individuals who have developed a concept of their bodies as hard and "tough." Such persons may have careers in the military, construction or other "hard edge" occupations. They depend on nicotine to numb their awareness and decrease both bodily and emotional sensitivity.

Snapdragon — Many people depend on the habit of putting a cigarette in the mouth as a substitute for food, or to curtail other "mouth energy" such as angry outbursts. Snapdragon helps redirect an over-abundance of fire in the mouth and throat (literally the practice of smoking) to other more healthy outlets in the metabolism and the emotions.

Chestnut Bud — For those who may have tried to quit many times and are stuck in a seemingly hopeless pattern of stopping and starting. Also helpful for ingrained habits and patterns that seek unconscious repetition in the act of smoking — such as the use of the hands, stimulation to the mouth when smoking, and so forth.

Social Smoke Screen: Cutting Ties that Bind

Walnut — Works with the client's determination to make the transition from an old lifestyle or identity to a new one — especially when there are many social cues, friends, family members or other circumstances that hypnotically entice the individual to have "one more smoke."

Goldenrod — This is a very important flower essence for those who do not have a well-developed individuality and smoke due to peer pressure, family rituals, or other forms of social conformity. It is especially helpful for adolescents who rebel against authority and adopt smoking as a "rite of passage," or as socially defiant gesture to set them apart.

Agrimony — For those who are attracted to tobacco in order to maintain a "cool" social exterior. Such individuals typically have emotional turmoil just beneath the surface of the personality, which they are able to keep "in control" through smoking.

Pink Monkeyflower — For those who are stuck in a cycle of shame or guilt about smoking, perhaps feeling that they are not "worth" recovery, or that they are hopelessly "bad." These soul feelings may be all the more acute if the individual is the only one at the workplace or in the family group who is smoking. Such individuals may have a deeper history of shock or abuse, resulting in an unconscious need to repeat such trauma by self-inflicting destructive behavior.

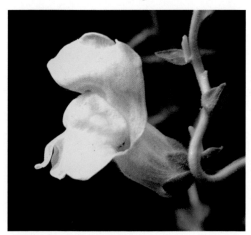

Snapdragon
Antirrhinum majus

Pink Monkeyflower
Mimulus lewisii

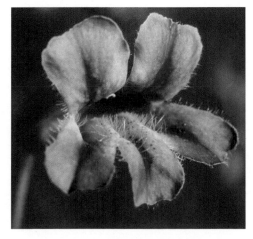

Nixing Nicotine: Detox Strategies

As any smoker knows, the hours, days and weeks following the last cigarette are the most intense and challenging — it is within this time period that the will to quit smoking can dissolve in an instant. Acute emotional states such as anxiety, tension, nervousness or depression can overwhelm the individual. At the same time, the body's self-cleansing efforts to rid itself of nicotine-related chemicals can result in toxic overload, with symptoms such as headaches, insomnia, acute lung congestion or purging, profound fatigue, or nausea. The following are strategies for coping with Nicotine Detox:

General Strategy — Breaking the cycle of any addiction is serious soul work. A time should be chosen when the individual is relatively free of major responsibilities or stress. Environmental triggers and social cues for smoking should be eliminated whenever possible (such as going to a party where old friends will be smoking). A support group of others who have overcome the same or similar addiction, and are willing to be called upon as needed, is very helpful. Enriching and stimulating activities such as nature walks, artistic projects, nourishing food and good literature or movies, should be planned in advance to give positive focus to this critical time period. Time should also be allowed for plenty of rest and quiet and for utilizing the detox procedures discussed below.

Prayer, Affirmation and Meditation — Breaking any addictive habit requires spiritual focus and soul wakefulness. Many individuals have found it helpful to create their own specialized prayers or affirmations, by evoking the positive qualities of the flower essences. This inner work is a powerful ally during moments of intense craving, encouraging the spiritual will to gain mastery over the lower will that is driven by desire. Combining flower essences with affirmation or prayer can create a potent synergy that increases the effectiveness of both modalities. It is also important to ask family and friends who have one's highest good in mind to help with prayer and other forms of positive support during the period of nicotine withdrawal.

Five-Flower Formula (or Rescue Remedy) — This is the single most important flower formula for coping with acute anxiety and other emotional symptoms resulting from nicotine withdrawal. Several drops can be taken directly from the stock bottle as often as needed, even hourly. A misting bottle containing Five-Flower Formula and other indicated flower essences can also be prepared. Many people find the misting method best for quick and convenient access.

Nicotiana — For intense bouts of nicotine craving take Nicotiana directly from the stock bottle as often as needed. It can also be combined with Five-Flower Formula for accompanying emotional anxiety.

Sagebrush and Sagebrush Smoke — Sagebrush flower essence addresses acute feelings of emptiness that arise when the individual is bereft of the drugs that have filled the inner space of the soul. Sagebrush flower essence is also very cleansing, eliminating both emotional and physical debris that clogs the system. Native American sagebrush smoke can be smudged around the aura for additional purification. This smudging ritual can also displace the acute need for smoking, by temporarily transferring the activity to another level.

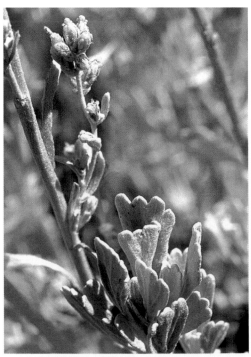

Sagebrush *Artemisia tridentata*

Self-Heal Detox Cream — One dropperful from the stock bottles of one or more of the four major flower essences profiled above — **Nicotiana, Yerba Santa, Morning Glory** and **Borage** — should be stirred into a base of **Self-Heal Creme**. Add to the cream four drops of pure Rose essential oil. This mixture should be massaged in a figure eight pattern (alternate in each direction) several times daily on the heart and chest region. When intense symptoms have subsided, the cream can be continued on a daily basis. This cream is very nourishing to the heart-lung region and will help to cleanse physical toxins as well as re-set the energetic receptors in this region of the body. Additional flower essences specific to the individual can also be added to the cream.

Detox Bath — Add two handfuls of Epsom salts and one handful of sea salt to a warm bath along with one dropperful each of **Nicotiana, Yerba Santa, Morning Glory, Borage** and **Sagebrush** flower essences. Stir the water in a figure eight pattern in each direction for about two minutes. Soak in the bath for approximately twenty minutes and then wrap in large towels for an additional twenty minutes. An alternative detox bath can be prepared with the same flower essences but, rather than salt, use clay (for example, Smoker's Detox Clay Bath from LL's Magnetic Clay). Either of these baths will pull toxic debris from the body. Many have reported the odor of tobacco following these baths, even several days after smoking cessation. During the intense phase of detox, this bath should be taken one or more times per day.

Detox Sweat — If there is access to a sauna, take **Sagebrush, Yerba Santa** and **Nicotiana** flower essences before, during and after a cleansing sweat. Also use several drops of Eucalyptus and Lemon essential oils to create a steam during the sauna to stimulate and cleanse the lungs. A smudge with Sagebrush smoke can also be used prior to, during, or after the sweat, if desired.

Another alternative is to make a strong tea from Sagebrush and/or Yarrow leaves. Strain the leaves and ladle the tea mixture onto the hot rocks during the sauna to create a gentle steam.

If the sweat is properly conducted it will be a time not only of physical detoxification, but also soul purification. Meditation and affirmation on the inner properties of the flower essences and the soul's goals for healing and change should be encouraged during this time.

If the sweat is properly conducted it will be a time not only of physical detoxification, but also soul purification.

Detox Facial Steam — To help break up congestion in the lungs, add two drops each of Eucalyptus and Lemon essential oils to a pan of hot steaming water. Add one dropperful of **Sagebrush** flower essence. Create a "hood" over the pan with towels and gently breathe in the steam mixture. A steam prepared from Sagebrush and Yarrow leaf tea can also be used in a similar manner. These procedures will relieve congestion in the lungs and speed the self-healing process.

Detox Precautions — It is necessary to drink ample amounts of water during any detox procedure. Also warm baths or saunas can alter potassium levels — so please seek professional nutritional advice. Finally, bathing, sweating or any other detoxification procedures may not be beneficial if there are medical contraindications. Please consult with a physician regarding your specific medical situation.

The Need for Nicotine: Deeper Soul Issues

Recovery from tobacco addiction is a significant achievement. However, many practitioners emphasize the need to explore wider healing themes, not always directly related to the nicotine addiction syndrome. Resolution of these issues frees the soul from the possibility of gravitating toward new addictive habits. While one can choose from the full spectrum of flower essences during this process, certain core healing themes are frequently involved.

The four primary flower essences for Nicotine Addiction discussed above (**Nicotiana, Yerba Santa, Borage** and **Morning Glory**) should be strongly considered as "anchors" when addressing the broader soul context. In addition, the following essences have been found helpful for issues arising out of emotional detox from addiction.

Light My Fire — Many individuals unconsciously gravitate toward smoking tobacco because of their need for fire, and for the masculine element in both the body and soul. Frequently, there is a deficiency in the relationship to the father, or in the ability to incorporate the masculine element in one's life (whether male or female). Essences which can be very beneficial in such cases include **Sunflower, Baby Blue Eyes, Poison Oak** and **Blazing Star**.

Tobacco becomes a crutch which gives a "false fire" or edge to the personality. The real task is to create that will power from within.

Empowering the Will — Related to the theme of the masculine self is the larger question of the will — the ability to focus one's attention and to manifest one's soul purpose in the world. Tobacco

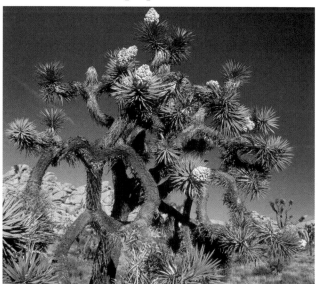

Joshua Tree is native to California's Mohave Desert. Clinical reports indicate that the Joshua Tree essence is excellent for breaking addictive patterns related to ones family or ethnic heritage.

becomes a crutch which gives a "false fire" or edge to the personality. The real task is to create that will power from within the soul itself. Flower essences that are indicated in such situations include **Blackberry, Cayenne, Wild Oat** and **Madia**.

Healing the Heart — The physical organ of the heart, and the energetic dynamics of the heart chakra, are the most severely affected by the use of tobacco. Very often there has been prior emotional trauma to the heart (or ongoing trauma) such as grief, rejection or abuse, which the individual continues to "cover" through nicotine addiction. In addition to **Yerba Santa, Borage,** and **Pink Monkeyflower** flower essences discussed above, the essences of **Bleeding Heart, Pink Yarrow, Holly, California Wild Rose, Love-Lies-Bleeding** or **Hawthorne** may be indicated in such circumstances, depending upon the specific soul trauma.

Growing Free on the Family Tree — Many people who smoke come from families of smokers, where lung cancer, emphysema, heart disease, and other smoker-related illnesses may be deeply embedded in the psychic and physical genetic code. Curiously, some individuals begin smoking after a loved one who is a smoker has died, as though the living link for the addiction is passed on to the next recipient. In addition to **Walnut** and **Goldenrod** flower essences discussed above, **Joshua Tree** essence is very beneficial for bringing the full consciousness of the family tree and hereditary karma to the awareness of the individual. Also important are the flower essences of **Red Clover, Mountain Pennyroyal, Yarrow** and **Angelica** to consolidate the energetic fields of those individuals who may be unconscious receptors for addictive patterns passed on from other family members, close friends, or lovers.

[1] There are 4000 different chemicals in cigarette smoke, including 43 that meet the stringent criteria for listing as known carcinogens. "Health Benefits of Smoking Cessation," 1990 Surgeon General report, as cited by David Moyer, MD, *The Tobacco Reference Guide*, 2000, available online at www.globalink.org/tobacco/org/

[2] CAN ("Clean Air Now," Dutch Non-Smoker's Association), Rotterdam, Netherlands, March, 1999, www.nietrokers.nl/e/denk4.html

Grounding Myself Without Tobacco:

A 27-Year Old Woman Develops her Own Soul Fire

A Case Report from Jyothi Rundel

The following article is a summary of a detailed case submitted to the **FES Certification Program** *by Wendy Jyothi Rundel. This outstanding report shows how "Meg" (not her real name) engages in a healing process through flower essence therapy. Meg overcomes her smoking addiction not simply by modifying her outer behavior, but by changing her soul identity. The flower essences awaken a new fire in Meg's soul that brings greater physical vitality, emotional equanimity and creative manifestation.*

A Background of Addiction

Meg initially sought flower essence therapy not only to cease smoking, but also to deal with troubling family circumstances that she suspected were at the core of her addiction.

Meg reported that many members of her family were afflicted with eating addictions, and that her father was an alcoholic who had a long-term affair with another woman while married to Meg's mother. She began smoking at age 21, when she was feeling isolated and under a great deal of stress while living abroad. She commented that with the family history of food addictions, she substituted smoking so that she would not get fat. Meg lived with a partner who also smoked, making it even harder to quit. Although generally healthy and still young, Meg showed signs of distress in her heart and chest — she tended to get sick from lung and bronchial flu, and pneumonia.

Meg was expressive about the deep pain she felt in her relationship with her father — as a traveling salesman he was frequently absent during her childhood and engaged in an extra-marital affair that brought much anguish to her mother. Meg's parents and other family lived a great distance away in the eastern United States. They had many expectations for her and disapproved of her current lifestyle and artistic aspirations. Her goal was to affirm her own unique identity and talents, especially to find renewed energy and inspiration for her career as an artist and photographer.

Primary Flower Essences

The following are the major flower essences used during therapy with Meg. These remedies were used in various formulas and at different intervals:

Nicotiana — To help Meg transform her addiction to nicotine, and reduce anxiety by giving her a positive, grounded relationship to her body and to the earth.

Sunflower — This was the core archetypal remedy that provided the foundation for Meg's healing, imparting positive masculine fire, and helping her soul build its own genuine forces of strength and solar radiance.

Baby Blue Eyes — To heal childhood wounds and vulnerabilities regarding Meg's relationship with her father.

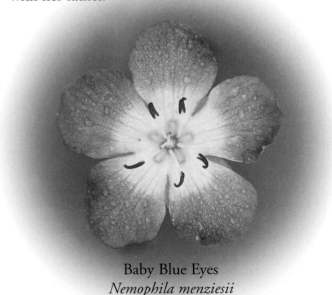

Baby Blue Eyes
Nemophila menziesii

Yerba Santa — To cleanse congestion in her heart and lungs both physically and emotionally; to help her bring expression to long-buried feelings and emotional wounds.

Pink Monkeyflower — To address the wounding in the heart region — to help Meg learn to take emotional risks with others, and to not "cover" her heart's emotions through nicotine addiction.

Chestnut Bud — To help break habitual patterns that contributed to her ongoing addiction to nicotine.

Blackberry — To bring new vitality to Meg's will forces; not only to heal her addiction to nicotine but to find new purpose and intention for her will forces.

Larch — To support a confident outlook on the world and to counteract doubt or hesitation, especially with regard to Meg's creative abilities.

Madia — To support Meg's focus on her new artistic goals and to overcome distraction or restlessness that could lead to resuming her old habit of tobacco.

Queen Anne's Lace — To integrate psychic, sexual and emotional energies in upper and lower chakras, and to bring new spiritual insight, vision and artistry to Meg's soul.

Iris — To open the creative portals of Meg's soul so that her true artistic talent and creativity could manifest with vibrancy and joy.

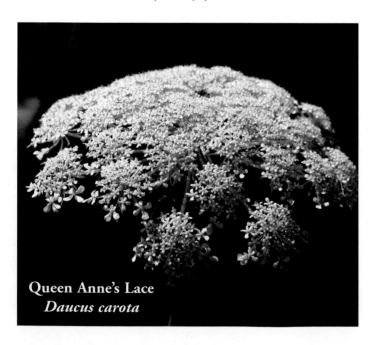

Queen Anne's Lace
Daucus carota

Uncovering "Deep Seated Pain and Emotion"

When Meg first began using flower essences, she noted that they "stirred up many deep seated pains and emotions which I was unconsciously aware I was harboring." Meg kept a very detailed journal which helped her to begin to understand and witness the new feelings that were surfacing. A core theme in her journal work involved her relationship with her father. She began to realize, "how the whole thing [with my father] had affected me, how I turned the resentment toward my father toward myself." These feelings were also being sorted out in relationship to her male partner.

After several months on flower essence therapy, Meg returned home to visit her parents. Meg had been absent one-and-a-half years and she was anxious about encountering her family. However, she reported that the "connections were clear, genuine and heartfelt … the flower essences helped me to maintain calmness, clarity and self-assurance."

Overcoming Nicotine Craving

During this same time period, Meg began to reduce her smoking. She used a stock bottle of **Nicotiana** to help her with intense bouts of craving, reporting that "the craving was not as annoying." Meg officially began her new business, reporting that she felt more confident and radiated more energy.

"I used tobacco for a loss of connection to the earth."

She then focused on a goal of complete smoking cessation. She frequently applied a cream mixture of flower essences directly to her heart and chest area (**Self-Heal Creme** with **Nicotiana, Yerba Santa**), along with stock doses of **Nicotiana** to offset specific cravings. A formula of **Nicotiana, Yerba Santa, Chestnut Bud, Queen Anne's Lace** and **Iris** was also used during this time period to provide emotional support and positive direction.

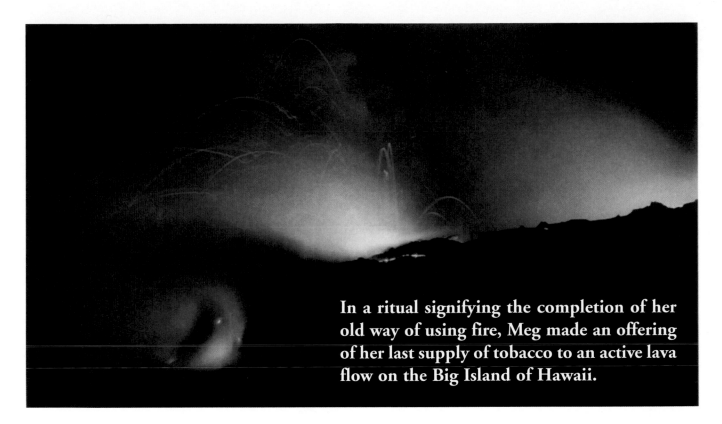

In a ritual signifying the completion of her old way of using fire, Meg made an offering of her last supply of tobacco to an active lava flow on the Big Island of Hawaii.

Bringing New Fire to Her Soul

After Meg had entirely quit smoking she noticed that her artwork was more vibrant and visionary. She also observed that her physical energy was more stable. "When I started smoking six years ago, I had a lot of energy … I am getting that energy back and making a fresh start. I didn't realize how ungrounded I was. I thought that's what the cigarettes were doing" [making her grounded].

"I can affirm that what I read of the research for the Nicotiana flower essence is true. I used tobacco for a loss of connection to the earth. I began smoking at age 21 when I was living in a city in Europe and drastically removed from nature," Meg wrote in her journal.

In a ritual signifying the completion of her old way of using fire, Meg made an offering of her last supply of tobacco to an active lava flow on the Big Island of Hawaii.

This act brought her into communion with the land that was now her home, and helped her to affirm a new way for her fire to be brought to the earth.

Follow-up: Meg has remained tobacco-free and the business which she founded to market her artistic products proved to be successful. Most importantly, she is healthy and radiant, and has given birth to her first child. Meg and her partner are enjoying being parents.

Wendy Jyothi Rundel was living in Kamuela, Hawaii, on the Big Island, at the time of this case. She currently resides in Oregon, where she practices Flower Essence Therapy, Jin Shin Tara and Craniosacral Therapy. She describes her intent as "empowering the client through inner awareness and self-healing." Jyothi welcomes your comments or contact at P.O. Box 42, Ashland, OR 97520, telephone 541-601-2683.

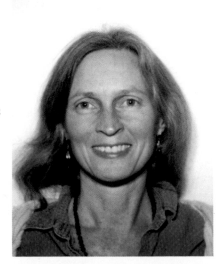

Tobacco:
From Sacred Plant to Addictive Drug

by Patricia Kaminski

Sacred Tobacco

It seems incredible to consider that in the course of just 500 years, a plant which had been considered as sacred and was used with great care in the religious ceremonies of countless Native American tribes, was subsequently transformed into a drug with devastating world-wide health consequences and extraordinary commercial profit.

Tobacco cultivation is estimated to be at least 10,000 years old. The native plants of *Nicotiana tabacum* and *Nicotiana rustica* were typically passed hand to hand from the slopes of the Andes Mountains in South America, north to the Great Plains and Great Lakes in North America. Rituals associated with tobacco were intended to help carry one's prayers to spiritual beings. They included the sprinkling of tobacco on fires in the sweat lodge, the offering of tobacco to the earth in various fertility ceremonies, and the creation of "medicine pouches," primarily featuring tobacco, that were worn over the heart-lung region.

The most elaborate ceremony involved smoking a ritual pipe, in which the participants offered tobacco in the four directions to create a common bond with each other and the earth, as a living being. The pipe ceremony was often the way in which conflict between tribes, or general tribal decision-making, was fostered.

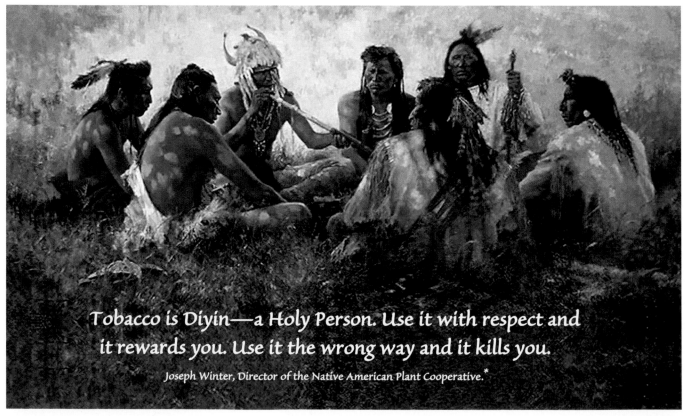

Tobacco is Diyin—a Holy Person. Use it with respect and it rewards you. Use it the wrong way and it kills you.

Joseph Winter, Director of the Native American Plant Cooperative.*

Crow Pipe Ceremony, art by Howard Terpning

> In ancient times, the land was barren and the people were starving. The Great Spirit sent forth a woman to save humanity. As she traveled over the world, everywhere her right hand touched the soil, there grew potatoes. And everywhere her left hand touched the soil, there grew corn. And when the world was rich and fertile, she sat down and rested. When she arose, there grew tobacco. — Native American Creation Story from the Huron Tribe

Many Native Americans believe that when tobacco began to be marketed as a vast commercial enterprise, dependent on southern plantation slave labor, its holy function was corrupted. As one tribal elder, White Deer of Autumn, explains, "The pipe is a link between the earth and the sky. Nothing is more sacred. The pipe is our prayer in physical form. Smoke becomes our words; it goes out, touches everything, and becomes a part of all there is. The fire in the pipe is the same fire in the sun, which is the source of life. You see what happens when a gift that has been given is misused. ... When a stem and bowl of the pipe are connected, you have a living being."

Profane Tobacco

After the European migration to the Americas, which began in 1492, tobacco was rapidly introduced throughout Europe: France in 1556, Portugal in 1558, Spain in 1559 and England in 1565. Jean Nico de Villemain, the French ambassador to Portugal, wrote about its medicinal properties in 1560 and the plant was eventually named for him. Commercial tobacco was processed in a manner that made it feel easier on the lungs, therefore enabling one to smoke it on a regular basis and thus become more easily addicted. The newly-created demand for nicotine products created a lucrative "cash crop," of incalculable benefit, especially to the American colonies.

Fueled by African slave labor, the United States quickly rose to a major world economic power, due in large measure to its tobacco plantations. The first Africans were brought into the state of Virginia around 1619, and in less than four decades, tobacco exports from Maryland and Virginia sextupled. Virgin land was replaced by tobacco fields as settlers moved westward and southward in an unrelenting drive. Tobacco became the economic lifeblood of the colonies and the means to exchange goods and services. By 1740, the Chesapeake Bay region was exporting 50% of the combined production of the world's tobacco-raising regions. Throughout the 17th and 18th centuries in America, tobacco was used as a monetary standard, lasting twice as long as the gold standard. A tobacco leaf was stamped upon the old Continental money used in the Revolution.

Over the centuries, tobacco was marketed in increasingly potent forms, from loose tobacco for pipes, to cigars, and finally to modern commercial cigarettes, featuring chemically laden "nicotine delivery systems." The sacred plant which had once been used for a peace pipe, was now used to create a hard edge for battlefield violence. Cigarettes were included as fundamental rations for the soldiers of both World Wars, and those opposing these measures where labeled "traitors." General John L. Pershing, commander of the American Expeditionary Force (AEF) in Europe during the First World War declared, "You ask me what we need to win this war. I answer tobacco as much as bullets. Tobacco is as indispensable as the daily ration; we must have thousands of tons without delay." During World War II, cigarettes were considered unofficial currency in Germany and valued at a minimum of 50 cents each.

Tobacco Addiction:
From World War to Madison Avenue

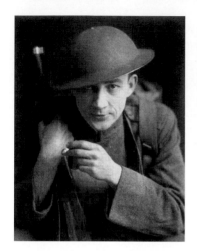

> "You ask me what we need to win this war. I answer tobacco as much as bullets."
>
> — General John L. Pershing, American commander in Europe, First World War

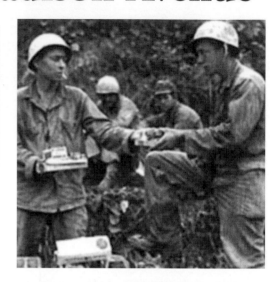

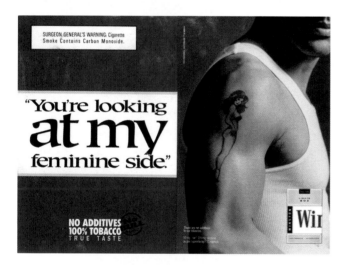

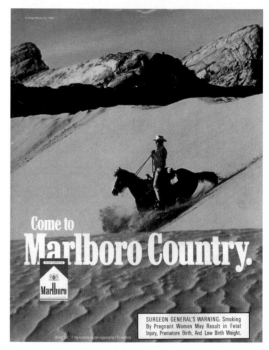

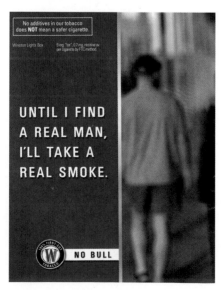

Advertisers continue to sell smoking and hard-edged masculinity.

> *Smoking was more of a way of rebelling than something I enjoyed. I thought I was cool and that it would make me more grown up like my parents who both smoked. I thought that my neighborhood pals would accept me if I joined the guys every day outside school to sneak a smoke. By the time I was in junior high, I was hooked on these deadly products, and I was willing to risk whatever future I might have had as a diver and an athlete, all to get my daily fix of those little tobacco sticks. ...*
>
> *Olympic Diver Greg Louganis as quoted in Merchants of Death by Larry C. White*

The manufacture and commercialization of tobacco reached a zenith right after World War II, with thousands of military personnel returning to their communities highly addicted and in turn, introducing countless others to tobacco. At the same time, extensive media advertising for tobacco products saturated all segments of society. By 1972, Reynolds Tobacco research scientist Claude Teague wrote, "The tobacco industry may be thought of as being a specialized, highly ritualized and stylized segment of the pharmaceutical industry. ... Happily for the tobacco industry, nicotine is both habituating and unique in its variety of physiological actions. ... "

* The Native American Plant Cooperative maintains a traditional tobacco seed bank, tobacco health education program, and tobacco leaf gift program, along with other Native American medicinal plants. Native American Plant Cooperative, P.O. Box 36749, Albuquerque, NM 87176.

References:

Borio, Gene, *The History of Tobacco*, http://www.historian.org/bysubject/tobacco1.htm

McGaa, Ed. *Mother Earth Spirituality: Native American Paths to Healing Ourselves and Our World*, HarperCollins, New York, NY: 1990.

Walter Reed Army Medical Center, *Brief History of Tobacco Use and Abuse*, http://www.wramc.amedd.army.mil/education/tobaccohistory.htm

White, Larry C., *Merchants of Death: The American Tobacco Industry*, Random House, New York, NY, 1988.

Other internet references:
www.usneighbor.org/native-american/pipe.htm
www.tobacco.org/History/Tobacco_History.html

> *To cease smoking is the easiest thing I ever did; I ought to know because I have done it a thousand times.*
>
> — Mark Twain

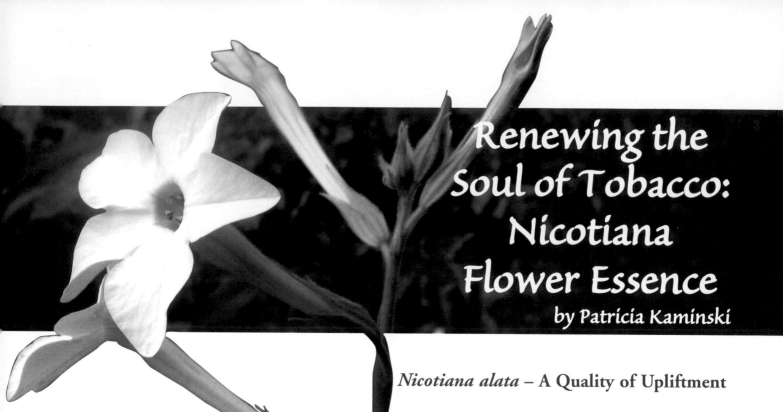

Renewing the Soul of Tobacco: Nicotiana Flower Essence
by Patricia Kaminski

Nicotiana alata – A Quality of Upliftment

Nicotiana alata is also known as "Flowering Tobacco," "Jasmine Tobacco" or "Night-Scented Tobacco." This species is native to the warm regions of South America and grows as a summer perennial in more temperate climates. The plant grows to about three feet (1 meter), and has tubular flowers that are typically white, although variations can be found in pink, red, and green flowers. (Nicotiana flower essence is made from the white-flowered varieties, although Green Nicotiana is also under research.)

Nicotiana alata is night blooming, with a rich, sweet fragrance that permeates the night air. The leaves are resinous and like its botanical relative, *Nicotiana tabacum*, the plant contains nicotine. It has some history of medicinal use as a masticatory herb because saliva is increased when it is chewed. The *N. alata* species has a gentle, airy quality; in fact, *alata* means "winged," and refers to the quality of the asymmetrical flowers seeming to take wing. While sharing characteristics of the traditional tobacco plant, it also has a unique quality that points to soul upliftment and transformation.

The Solanaceae Plant Family

Nicotiana is a member of the **Solanaceae** botanical plant family, also known as **Nightshades**. This extensive plant family contains many species native to the Americas, particularly edible foods such as peppers, tomatoes, eggplant and potatoes. It also contains many plants which are poisonous due to powerful alkaloids, such as Belladonna and Datura.

The poisonous members of this family can be important medicines. Many notable homeopathic remedies are made from the most toxic members of the Solanaceae plants, including *Datura stramonium* (Jimson Weed) for terror and fear, *Atropa belladonna* (Belladonna) for violent tendencies, *Mandragora officinalis* (Mandrake) for manic-depressive episodes, *Hyocyamus niger* (Henbane) for wild and inflated behaviors. These same four plants were also used in medieval occult ritual to stimulate astral consciousness, such as the ability to fly in dreams. In homeopathic medicine, this family of plants addresses intense, typically covert psychic forces that may paralyze or overwhelm the consciousness.

Darkness and Interior Light

FES research into three members of the Solanaceae family points to a further refinement of these basic themes, when prepared as flower essences. It is significant that the two most common names for the entire plant family refer to opposite qualities – **Solanaceae** indicates a fire quality that is related to, or is like the sun (**sol**). **Nightshade** refers to the propensity of this family to bloom at night, or to be stimulated by darkness (such as potato heads that are able to sprout in darkness without any orientation to the sun). These seeming opposites can be integrated as one archetypal wholeness if we consider the manner in which darkness can be illumined by an interior light of the soul, a light which is not the external sun, but shines as the sun would.

The **Angel's Trumpet** (*Brugmansia candida*) flower essence helps the soul transcend fear of the unknown at the time of dying, by learning to trust the light of interior consciousness. **Cayenne** (*Capsicum annum*) flower essence stimulates a part of the lethargic will that is clouded and opaque to higher consciousness. *Nicotiana alata* lights an interior fire, especially in the region of the heart and lung, and its relationship to the metabolic will. It is a quality that is both grounding and stimulating, helping the will to cultivate a calm and focused energy state that is infused with life force.

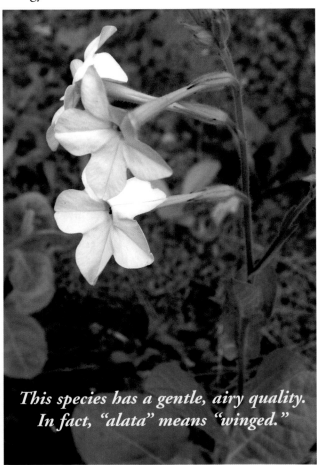

This species has a gentle, airy quality. In fact, "alata" means "winged."

The Heart of the Living Earth and the Human Heart

Nicotiana flower essence heals the craving for the false fire of metabolic arousal through tobacco addiction. Quite literally, the use of tobacco increases the physical heart rate, while anesthetizing and numbing the feelings of the heart. Life is felt more intensely as a sense of personal power and bodily stimulation, rather than as a relationship with a matrix of nurturing forces.

While Nicotiana flower essence can be beneficial for tobacco addiction, it also speaks to a general *dis-ease* that challenges the contemporary soul living in a technological culture. Native American sacred tobacco ritual aligned the human heart with the life pulsation or "drumbeat" of the living Earth. The user of the peace pipe felt the interior reality or "heart" of Mother Earth, creating a transcendent consciousness in the body and soul.

In modern culture, the genuine heartbeat of the earth is distorted in an automated, technological society that is hyper-stimulated, and out of touch with the natural rhythms of life. Surrender to the true healing powers of the night through sleep and a cadenced lifestyle are bypassed in favor of hyper-will force, artificially roused through electrical light and a host of mechanized conveniences and stimulants. As a result, both body and soul are compressed and hardened into an intense and isolated form of ego consciousness. At its extreme, the false macho persona of the "Marlboro man" uses the drumbeat of the living Earth for the drumbeat of industrial war, eco-violence and extreme power divorced from feelings. A living relationship to the rhythms of Earth and to the interior feminine light of the soul has been transformed into its very opposite.

Nicotiana flower essence helps the heart find *life fire,* which is not divorced from *soul feelings.* The flower essence of Nicotiana re-instills the true spiritual teaching of the tobacco plant: radiant peace arises from being able to access the deep life chamber of the heart and through the path of the heart, find connection to the Earth and all living beings.

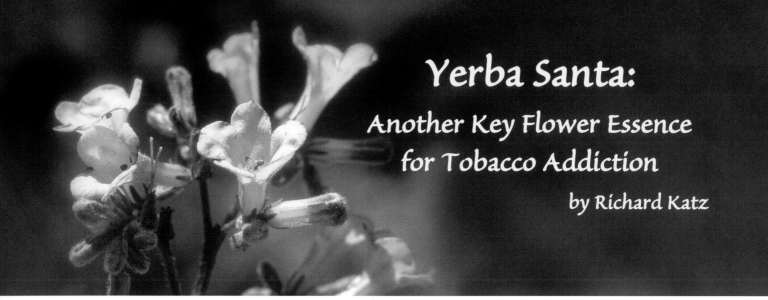

Yerba Santa:
Another Key Flower Essence for Tobacco Addiction
by Richard Katz

The common names of Yerba Santa (*Eriodictyon californicum*) include Mountain Balm, Bear's Weed, Gum Plant, Consumptive Weed, and Sacred Herb. It was used medicinally by Native American healers for many centuries, and then taken up by the Spanish settlers, who gave it its current name, meaning "Holy Herb."

Yerba Santa flower essence is indicated for those who hold in the water element, especially manifest in the emotions of grief, melancholy, depression or despair.

Yerba Santa is an evergreen aromatic shrub with woody rhizomes, typically growing to a height of 3 to 4 feet (1m +). The dark green, leathery leaves are oblong to lanceolate and covered with shiny resin. They grow in an alternate arrangement and are pinnately veined and usually serrated. The taste of the leaves is balsamic and the flowers and leaves smell pleasantly aromatic on a warm day. Yerba Santa is native to the western and southwestern regions of North America, and is somewhat native to northern Mexico. It grows 2-6 feet (0.6 to 2 m) in height at elevations ranging from 2,000 to 3,500 feet (600 to 1000 m). It is typically found in dry areas that are sparse of other vegetation. The flowers are a delicate whitish-lavender color, found in curved tubular clusters (helicoid cymes) at the top of the plant, and are pollinated by butterflies.

Yerba Santa blooms from May to July, depending on the elevation. The fruit forms a grayish-brown seed capsule, oval in shape, which contains hardened black seeds.

Yerba Santa is an exceptional member of the Waterleaf Family (Hydrophyllaceae) which also contains Phacelia, Baby Blue Eyes and Fiesta Flower. Most of these family members grow in cool, moist habitats, indicating a strong relationship to the watery element. Yerba Santa also has a relationship with water, although in an opposite way. With its tough, resinous leaves, it holds and conserves its water from the inside to meet the intense fire of its environment. This quality helps us to understand the medicinal use of Yerba Santa as a regulator of the water element. Yerba Santa coats the mucous membranes and holds the aqueous component in contact with the cells, re-establishing mucopolysaccharides. As such, it is an excellent herbal remedy for chronic respiratory ailments, used as an expectorant to treat coughs and congestion, as well as aiding in loosening and expelling phlegm. It dilates bronchial tubes, and thus is used to ease asthma and allergy attacks. A tea, tincture or syrup is typically made from the leaves, sometimes including the flowers. Smoke from the leaves may be used as well.

A picture of the soul qualities of the Yerba Santa essence emerges from this botanical herbal portrait. Yerba Santa flower essence is indicated for those who hold in the water element, especially manifest in the emotions of grief, melancholy, depression or despair. These emotions are stored in the deeper cavities of the body, particularly in the heart/lung/respiratory region. The free flowing, or "breathing out," of soul expression is often impeded. Respiratory illnesses, addiction to tobacco, and various allergies are common physical manifestations of this soul imbalance.

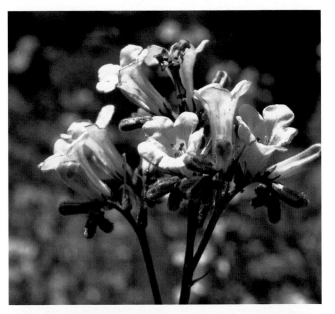

Yerba Santa frees the lungs and heart to acknowledge and release stored emotional experiences. Yerba Santa was regarded as a holy herb by the native peoples, because the process of awakening, and claiming deep soul experience leads to an indwelling "Temple of the Spiritual Self." It is often in those places where the soul retains the most profound pain or trauma, that the strongest teachings of the Spiritual Self can also be realized.

The color and form of the Yerba Santa is truly a signature of these soul qualities—the delicate lavender flowers suggest a highly refined level of spiritual awareness. And at the same time the curving, tubular shaped flowers speak to a process of descent into the deepest parts of the soul temple. The insights of Matthew Wood, in *Seven Herbs Plants as Teachers* capture in a most touching way, these qualities of Yerba Santa:

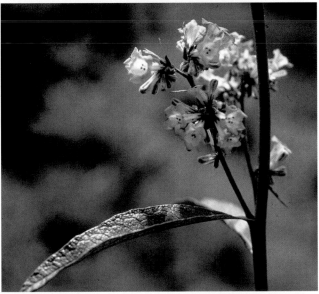

> *"The inner spaces defined by the body lining are 'sanctuaries,' from which impurities must be kept. Perhaps it was an intuitive recognition of this which gave the plant its name: Yerba Santa ... the internal body linings correspond with "psychic body linings." Sanctity of psychic space is the internal property which Yerba Santa guards."*
>
> Matthew Wood

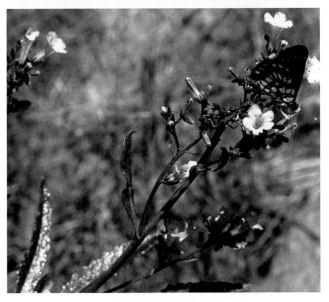

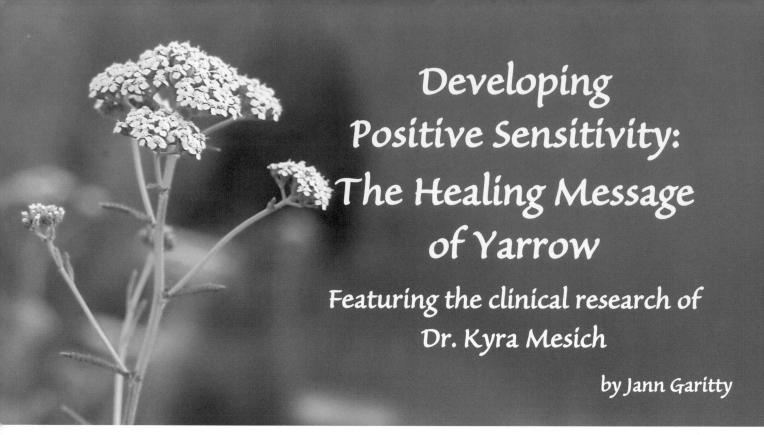

Developing Positive Sensitivity: The Healing Message of Yarrow

Featuring the clinical research of Dr. Kyra Mesich

by Jann Garitty

The Challenge of Sensitivity

For sensitive individuals, life can be excruciatingly painful, with daily events and relationships severely limited or disrupted. The dynamic of sensitivity and empathy manifests in two polarities: *inward receptivity* for registering psychic information and *outward projection* through merging unconsciously with others. Each modality has the potential to trigger inappropriate or maladaptive emotions or behaviors.

Sensitivity and empathy can create social and psychological complications. Overly sensitive individuals may lose self-awareness in relationships, due to an overwhelm of emotions and information, even to the point of not knowing their own opinions, likes or dislikes. Those with additional societal disadvantages (children or adults with learning disabilities, for example) are further compromised if they are vulnerable, highly sensitive or empathic.

In many societies, highly developed perceptive or "psychic" abilities are not given validation. Hence, individuals with these abilities may feel isolated or marginalized. If such a person has not learned to embrace the capacity for intense receptivity in a conscious, positive manner, others may view them as having a weak or debilitating condition. This perception is reinforced by the fact that some sensitives are indeed often not able to cope well and are easily distressed. Additionally, they may suffer from guilt, blaming themselves for the difficulties they experience with others and the world around them. In response to their difficulties, and lack of understanding by others, they may act out inappropriate behaviors, have feelings of low self-esteem or experience anxiety or depression.

Sensitivity: An Asset, Not a Liability

Individuals who are empathic or sensitive can transform the debilitating effects described above into beneficial assets and strengths that contribute to well-being. Psycho-spiritual practices, such as meditation and visualization, can aid individuals in establishing a clear separation between themselves and incoming energetic stimulation from other people or the environment. When kept in balance, the capacity of acute perception is a valuable tool for deepening one's experiences of the world. The richness of such perception can bring great joy and meaning to one's life.

The various Yarrow flower essences have proven to be effective in helping "sensitives" with acute psychic perception and heightened empathic abilities. These individuals may have difficulty with their psychic boundaries in relationships. Dr. Kyra Mesich's research about psychic sensitivity validates the important contribution of the Yarrow flower essences.

The Research of Dr. Mesich

Dr. Kyra Mesich, a clinical psychologist in Minneapolis, Minnesota, is a pioneering researcher and teacher in the field of empathy and psychic sensitivity. She has collected considerable case research on empathic ability, which she defines as "the capacity to literally feel another person's emotional experience." She also recognizes that these problems are exacerbated due to our society's denial and repression of the existence of psychic phenomena.

According to Dr. Mesich, "The biggest question sensitive people have is, 'why.'" Why are they so sensitive, why do they react so differently to the world than the "average" person? In *The Sensitive Person's Survival Guide,* Dr. Mesich provides answers to this question, along with insights and practices that can help the sensitive person. She believes that the Yarrow flower essences are a crucial component in dealing with sensitivity and general empathic ability.

The Energetic Field

Dr. Mesich's research corroborates the empirical evidence gathered by the *Flower Essence Society*, showing that the various Yarrow flower essences help provide a *protective shield* against potentially harmful sensations, over-stimulation, and merging with others. To understand why this is true, it is helpful to look at the phenomena of sensitivity and empathic ability in relation to the *energetic body.*

If we wish to move beyond a completely materialistic conception of life, it is essential to recognize that all living beings are enveloped by a permeable energy field called the *aura.* In some instances, the aura may be too porous, or have gaps, creating an inflow of external psychic information that can be overwhelming. Additionally, the auric field is dynamic and has the capacity to merge outwardly with one's surroundings and with the other psychic fields. Ideally, the aura should regulate the energy it accepts and emits, with a filtering function to protect the individual's well-being, and core sense of Self. Thus, the aura is similar to the physical circulatory system, regulating an inflow and outflow of psychic information.

Yarrow: A Shield of Protection

Observing the Yarrow plant (*Achillea millefolium*), we see the open, feather-like structure of the leaves, and the mass of tiny individual flowers that form a contiguous structure. Both the leaves and flowers include a multitude of finely articulated structures that form a gestalt, suggesting both protection and permeability.

Yarrow herb is well known within herbal tradition for its vulnerary and astringent properties — literally able to staunch wounds and control bleeding — with old names like Soldier's Wound

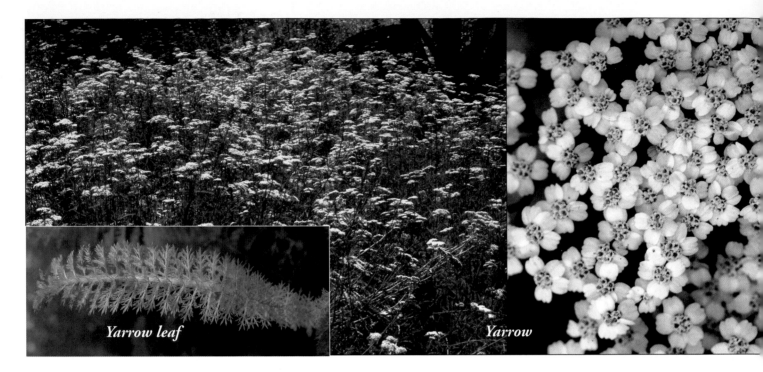

Yarrow leaf

Yarrow

Wort and Knight's Milfoil, or Herba Militaris. Herbal legend associates the plant with the Greek warrior, Achilles, who was brave in battle despite his vulnerable "Achilles heel." It is from this association that the genus name, *Achillea*, derives.

The Yarrow flower essence works on a psychic level to heal the bleeding or merging of the aura with the surrounding emotional environment. As Dr. Mesich writes in her book, "Just as the herbal Yarrow cleanses and heals the skin after a wound, Yarrow essence heals and rebalances the empathetic person's energetic boundaries and natural empathic protection."

Herbal tradition also describes how Yarrow not only stops bleeding, but in certain circumstances, can also stimulate bleeding. (Yarrow was called "Nose Bleed," but also "Staunchweed." See note on page 157.) Therefore we can say, it *regulates* bleeding. It breaks up clots and thins the blood, but it also acts as an astringent to control bleeding.

The Yarrow flowers are very important to our modern world. All people have been wounded by living in a technological world that emphasizes materialism, narrow intellectualism, and a cacophony of sensory experiences. For some people, this causes psychic stress, or bleeding, and for others, the result is stagnation and hardening. Yarrow

flower essence circulates and regulates the energetic expression of the aura in a manner similar to the Yarrow's herbal function in regulating the circulation of blood.

A Spectrum of Yarrow Essences

Flower essences are made from three different Yarrow plants: *Achillea millefolium* is the common white Yarrow that grows wild throughout the temperate regions of the world. *Achillea millefolium* var. *rubra*, is a variety known as Pink Yarrow. The pale pink variety occurs naturally, and a deeper pink cultivar is used for the flower essence. *Achillea filipendulina* is a more robust species known as Golden Yarrow. Named for its dense head of golden yellow flowers, it is also called "Fernleaf Yarrow." A fourth Yarrow remedy is a composite formula, *Yarrow Environmental Solution*, which includes the three Yarrow essences, plus Arnica and Echinacea, along with Yarrow and Echinacea tinctures and Celtic Sea Salt.

The ongoing research of the *Flower Essence Society* and the specific research of Dr. Mesich shows that the different Yarrow essences address specific aspects of sensitivity:

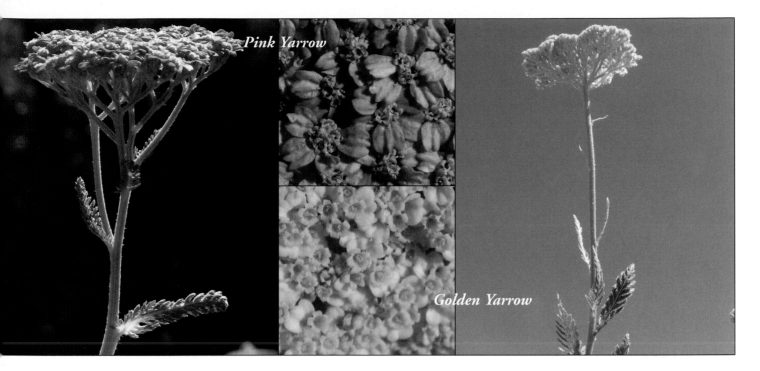

Pink Yarrow

Golden Yarrow

Pink Yarrow

❖ imparts strong grounding and vitalizing forces
❖ fosters emotional cohesion for those who merge too easily with their psychic environment

Pink Yarrow people:

❖ lack a confident sense of self and look to complete themselves in relationship to other people
❖ are often involved in relationships where they "give too much"
❖ attempt to solve people's problems so they won't have to feel the pain of others
❖ typically have grown up in chaotic or abusive families without emotional support

Golden Yarrow

❖ self-protection for those who feel vulnerable about creative expression and communication
❖ particularly helpful for artists, actors and others who combine sensitivity with social responsibilities

Golden Yarrow people:

❖ attempt to build barriers of protection
❖ may be involved in artistic or demanding social professions
❖ may withdraw from the world or appear timid, shy, cold
❖ create boundaries between themselves and the emotional pain they feel as empathics, including the possibility of drug abuse

Yarrow (White)

❖ a multi-purpose remedy for the age and time we live in, with benefits beyond the personal sensitivities discussed above

White Yarrow people:

❖ experience various forms of sensitivity or are not sure what direction their sensitivity takes
❖ tend to absorb and process their sensitivity in the higher mental fields, as distinct from the personal emotional sensitivity of the Pink Yarrow type

Yarrow Environmental Solution

(previously known as Yarrow Special Formula)

❖ designed to help the body cope with geopathic stress — such as radiation, electromagnetic fields and various toxic substances
❖ helpful for those whose sensitivity has somatized into various physical illnesses, such as allergies or chemical sensitivities
❖ an excellent remedy for strengthening the immune system but not as specific for various forms of psychic sensitivity and internalized soul conditions

Healing the Wounded Healer

Dr. Mesich feels that meditation practice and psychic training are important tools for sensitives. She points out that sensitive people are already naturally gifted, and can benefit from learning how to use this ability skillfully. "Yarrow is the remedy of the wounded warrior, but these days it's the remedy for the wounded healer," she writes. When referring to healers, she includes nurses, doctors, and health practitioners, as well as teachers, lawyers, and counselors — all people who are involved in social professions that demand sensitive perception and social acuity.

Dr. Mesich wrote *The Sensitive Person's Survival Guide* out of her own experience as a "wounded healer." Despite her extensive training to become a clinical psychologist, she received absolutely no information about the energetic manifestation of emotions. She was trained to have clear separation between patients and her personal life, but came to realize these abstract intellectual structures were meaningless without an understanding of energetic boundaries. Professionals receive concentrated training in their specific field of work, but there's a considerable lack of information about the actual psychic dynamics of empathy and sensitivity. With additional understanding and experience, professionals could perform without being drained and personally hurt. They would be able to give from a stable psychic center, and help their clients more effectively.

Working with Environmental Sensitives

Since writing her book, Dr. Mesich has been contacted by many people who are physically and chemically sensitive individuals. This has impelled her to consider the healing context for people with physical sensitivity. Due to heightened sensitivity and painful reactions to many substances, these individuals hesitate to use flower essences. Rather than internal dosages, Dr. Mesich recommends topical applications, holding the essence in the hand, or misting the essence in one's environment.

About Dr. Kyra Mesich

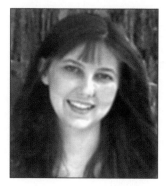

Kyra Mesich, Psy.D., earned her doctoral degree in clinical psychology from the Florida Institute of Technology's APA-approved program in Melbourne, Florida. In the years since her training, Dr. Mesich has studied extensively in the field of alternative health, including herbalism, flower essence therapy, energy healing and meditation. Dr. Mesich is the author of *The Sensitive Person's Survival Guide*, and winner of the 2000 Innovation Award from the Small Publishers Association of North America. She works and resides in Minneapolis, Minnesota. Please visit her website: www.KyraMesich.com

About Jann Garitty

Jann is a vital part of the FES staff, involved with writing, research and practitioner outreach. She has a wide variety of interests and commitments as a jeweler, gardener and herbalist. For over 30 years, she has worked with Native American organizations in education, arts, and cultural outreach and has served as the Director of the Sierra Storytelling Festival. Jann is the mother of two grown children and lives in the Sierra Nevada foothills of northern California with her husband and a menagerie of animal companions.

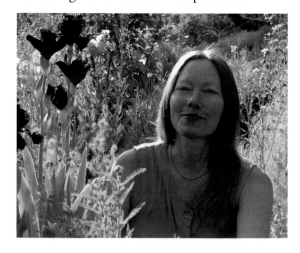

Golden Yarrow for Sensitivity & Self Integrity

by Kyra Mesich, Psy.D.

The following two cases demonstrate how Golden Yarrow flower essence can have a profound impact on the varied symptoms that accompany the sensitive personality. Doug, an adult male with chronic depressive episodes, and Ruthie, a young child diagnosed with ADD, both benefited from a new approach to their sensitivity, including the use of Golden Yarrow essence.

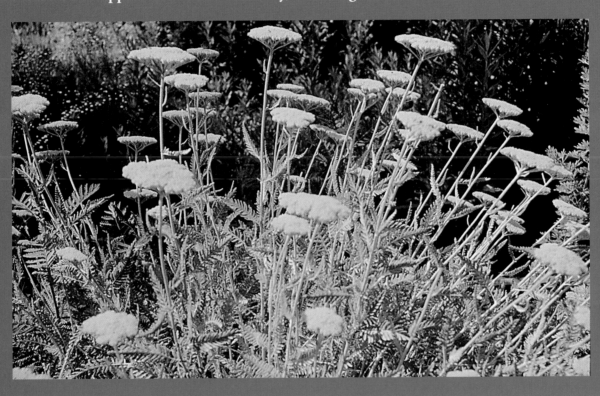

Doug:
A Case of Recalcitrant Depression

Doug is a 37-year old married man. He is very tall, attractive and healthy in appearance. He reports that he comes from an artistic, yet conservative family. His parents are artists, but his father was also a church pastor. Doug has worked professionally as a musician and appears to have inherited his parents' creative multi-talents.

Doug's primary concerns included a lack of direction in his career, chronic depressive episodes, and spontaneous psychic experiences. Doug described that several times a year he is overcome with severe depression, which can be incapacitat-

ing and last for up to three to four weeks. Doug is naturally intuitive, and admits to varied psychic experiences, which he has rarely discussed with anybody. He describes himself as a sensitive person, with an emotional nature, empathic understanding of others, artistic abilities, and a tendency to feel overwhelmed by stressors or social interaction.

His interest in sensitivity led him to read *The Sensitive Persons Survival Guide*. Based on the information about flower essences learned from the book, Doug identified with Golden Yarrow. He began taking Golden Yarrow essence and reported a change in the experience of his depressive episodes after consistent use during a period of two weeks. Subsequently, he stated that he felt a depressive episode coming on, and was expecting the typical two week incapacitation. Instead, he found that he was able to work through the depression in a matter of two hours — an experience he had never had prior to taking the Golden Yarrow flower essence.

Doug explained that he was not overcome by the usual depressive thoughts and moods. He was able to maintain some emotional objectivity while doing journal writing and talking with his wife. After a couple of hours, he felt the dark mood lift. Doug reported this experience with much surprise and enthusiasm.

He found that he was able to work through the depression in a matter of two hours — an experience he had never had prior to taking the Golden Yarrow flower essence.

Since using Golden Yarrow flower essence, Doug noted the following emotional shifts: his sensitivity did not seem as intense — he could be around groups of people or moderately stressful situations without feeling overwhelmed. He felt more hopeful about his career future. He began to connect his creative talents and intuitive abilities in ways he had not considered before, such as new ideas for writing and music projects.

Additional Note: The Golden Yarrow flower essence did not completely eliminate Doug's depression, nor did it numb him to his emotional experiences. To the contrary, the result appeared to be a greater synthesis of his emotions, abilities and sense of self. Doug enrolled in a course of classes to develop his intuitive and psychic abilities. Benefits from the classes and Golden Yarrow flower essence left Doug with a greater feeling of control over his sensitivities, and a better understanding of how his gifts and talents can be used in his career and life. He continues to experience a significantly reduced intensity of depressive episodes, during which he is now able to look inward and gain a greater understanding of himself, rather than completely shutting down in pain as before.

Ruthie: A Complex Case of Behavioral Problems

At the time this case was conducted, Ruthie was a seven-year old girl, enrolled in second grade public school. She has one younger brother, and three older siblings. Her parents divorced when she was 8 months old. Her mother has since remarried. Ruthie lives with her mother and siblings. She has regular visits with her biological father.

The mother contacted the author for a consultation with the following concerns: Ruthie had continual behavioral problems at school, including acting out, stealing items and poor completion of schoolwork. At home, Ruthie's behavioral problems continued with frequent arguments with siblings and tantrums. The mother described that Ruthie seemed to lack an understanding of social relationships and boundaries. Because of Ruthie's numerous behavioral problems at school, she has been diagnosed with Attention Deficit Disorder by a school psychologist.

Ruthie's mother wasn't satisfied with the ADD diagnosis as an explanation of Ruthie's behavior, and wanted to gain a better understanding of the underlying issues resulting in Ruthie's numerous problems. The mother described that Ruthie's behavior seemed at its worst when Ruthie was at the center of attention. For example, when singled out in class to answer a question or engage in an activity, Ruthie would react erratically with developmentally inappropriate responses (as if she was three years old, according to her mother). This trend continued at home, where Ruthie would respond to direct attention from siblings or parents with aggressive behavior or with tantrums.

Ruthie's mother surmised that she began seeing behavioral changes in her daughter when she was two years old. At that time, Ruthie seemed to undergo a personality change from a personable baby to a moody, withdrawn, and sometimes spacey toddler. The mother admitted that she had tried numerous venues to help Ruthie with no success. She said that her biggest concern was that she couldn't understand Ruthie. She explained further that she appreciated the motivations and behavior of her other four children but didn't feel connected to Ruthie, and was at a loss to know how to help her.

Ruthie's symptom picture was fairly severe. Because of the complexity of Ruthie's case, treatment began with a healing session to uncover the origins of her dysfunction. Golden Yarrow was identified as a key flower essence. Ruthie's behavioral problems primarily stemmed from her reaction to her parents' divorce. The personality change emerged at age two when Ruthie became developmentally able to have cognitive understanding of what the divorce meant for her family. Ruthie reacted by feeling her world had fallen apart. She responded by testing the boundaries of family, school and social interactions.

She felt vulnerable and emotionally shattered following her parents' divorce. ... Golden Yarrow honed in on the core issues of vulnerability and social disconnection.

Although Ruthie did not appear as a typically sensitive child, this was exactly the area where she needed the greatest support. She felt vulnerable and emotionally shattered following her parents' divorce. This affected her sense of self and her ability to trust or connect with anyone, adult or peer. Golden Yarrow honed in on the core issues of vulnerability and social disconnection.

Ruthie responded positively to healing interventions, including Golden Yarrow. For example, her mother was stunned to report that for the first time ever, Ruthie apologized to one of her siblings following an argument. The mother reported that Ruthie had never before exhibited such socially appropriate behavior of her own accord. This instance was followed by other small steps which demonstrated that Ruthie was cautiously but steadily reconnecting with the people around her.

(Please note that the author is keenly aware that in childhood cases of disruptive behavioral outbursts and/or personality changes; sexual, emotional and physical abuse should always be investigated as possible causes. These factors were investigated and ruled out.)

In summary, these two cases demonstrate the powerful benefits that Golden Yarrow essence can have toward apparently overwhelming psychological problems. These cases also show how sensitivity can manifest quite differently by age group. In straightforward cases, adults will self-identify as a sensitive personality type. Children, on the other hand, typically cannot self-report their inner experiences. It is not uncommon that a young child's response to social overwhelm culminates in inappropriate behavioral outbursts. It is likely that without intervention, Ruthie would have grown up to be an easily identifiable Golden Yarrow type, prone to social isolation, oversensitivity, or substance abuse. Despite their differences, both these cases evidenced the core meaning of Golden Yarrow: to bring forth integrity of the self in a social context.

End Note

Wood, Matthew, *The Book of Herbal Wisdom*, North Atlantic Books, Berkeley, California, 1997. See page 68, where Wood references John Gerard (1597) and Maude Grieve (1931).

The Flower Essence Society

A Quarter Century of International Research and Education

The *Flower Essence Society* is an international network of flower essence practitioners, researchers, and educators. Your membership and donations keep you in touch with the latest developments in flower essence therapy. Through your generous support, the *Flower Essence Society* is able to continue its plant study and clinical research, develop in-depth educational programs, grant scholarships to practitioners working with disadvantaged populations and facilitate our worldwide networking effort.

Education: training and certification programs for flower essence practitioners throughout the world.

Publications: books, booklets, e-newsletters, *Calix* journal, and a rich spectrum of clinical reports and practitioner profiles on our web site.

International Networking: a communication network for those who are teaching, researching or practicing in the field of flower essence therapy, including the FES online Practitioner Referral Network.

Research: Botanical studies of flower essence plants, empirical clinical research, practitioner surveys and scientific studies.

Visit our web site at www.flowersociety.org to learn more!

Membership has it benefits!

... *access to our exclusive Members' Pages*
    featuring profiles of our FES research essences

... *access to our updated, full-color online Repertory (for members only)*
    now with color plant photos and interactive selection guide

... *FES Members' Email Newsletter with practitioner reports, case studies,*
    scientific research, plant profiles, book reviews, class announcements

... *the opportunity to join the FES Practitioner Referral Network*
    help clients find you online with a user-friendly, searchable database

... *Calix: International Journal of Flower Essence Therapy*
    the next full-color volume sent to all members when published

---

Join the Flower Essence Society Now

"I offer my highest praise to the **Flower Essence Society**. Your educational work with therapists all over the world, and commitment to high-quality research, produces a level of professionalism that is unparalleled in the flower essence community."

Dr. Claudia Stern, Director, Centro de Estudios Florales y Naturales, Buenos Aires, Argentina

Name _____

Address _____

_____

Telephone _____ Fax _____ E-mail: _____

Professional affiliation _____

Description of your health practice and use of flower essences _____

_____

Research interests and other comments _____

_____

_____

Choose one of the following Membership Categories

❏ **Flower** Individual — $25 per year: basic level of support ($30 outside North America)

❏ **Bouquet** Organizational — $50 per year: for organizations and stores

❏ **Garden** Supporting — $100 per year: assists education & research

❏ **Garden Angel** Lifetime — $500: a life-long association with our work

❏ **Heart Blossom**: I am enclosing $_____ as an additional donation to support the educational and research work of Earth-Spirit, Inc. (tax-deductible in the US: IRS# 94-2804926). Please apply it to:

    ❏ Any program of the Society   ❏ Educational programs and scholarships
    ❏ Research programs   ❏ Publications

Total amount $_____ ❏ Check enclosed

❏ Please charge my Visa / MasterCard / Discover / American Express

Card number _____ Expiration _____

Cardholder name _____

Signature _____

You can also sign-up online, or by telephone or fax:

Flower Essence Society, P.O. Box 459, Nevada City, CA 95959 USA
800-736-9222   530-265-9163   fax: 530-265-0584
mail@flowersociety.org   www.flowersociety.org

Flowers are beautiful
hieroglyphics of Nature,
with which she indicates
how much she loves us.
— Johann von Goethe

Lotus *Nelumbo nucifera*